LOOK YOUNGER, LIVE LONGER

LOOK *Younger*

LIVE *Longer*

BY GAYELORD HAUSER

FARRAR, STRAUS
AND COMPANY : NEW YORK

FIRST PRINTING, FEBRUARY, 1950
SECOND PRINTING, MARCH, 1950
THIRD PRINTING, MAY, 1950
FOURTH PRINTING, JUNE, 1950
FIFTH PRINTING, JULY, 1950
SIXTH PRINTING, AUGUST, 1950
SEVENTH PRINTING, OCTOBER, 1950
EIGHTH PRINTING, OCTOBER, 1950
NINTH PRINTING, OCTOBER, 1950
TENTH PRINTING, OCTOBER, 1950
ELEVENTH PRINTING, OCTOBER, 1950
TWELFTH PRINTING, NOVEMBER, 1950
FOURTEENTH PRINTING, NOVEMBER, 1950
FIFTEENTH PRINTING, DECEMBER, 1950

For Lady Mendl, who long ago did
what *I hope every reader of this book will do:*
She fell in love with life.

TABLE OF CONTENTS

SECTION ONE : YOUR GOOD HEALTH

vii

SECTION TWO : YOUR GOOD LOOKS

SECTION THREE : YOUR GOOD LIFE

LOOK YOUNGER, LIVE LONGER DIET PLAN

SECTION ONE

YOUR GOOD HEALTH

I. PASSPORT TO A NEW WAY OF LIFE

YOU ARE making a mistake.

Just now, you began reading a book. It is in your hands: a book by Gayelord Hauser, entitled *Look Younger, Live Longer*. You intend to read this book like any other book. Like a magazine or detective story.

That is your mistake.

The book in your hands is no ordinary book. You are holding a passport to a new way of living. You are not just beginning to read. You are beginning a new adventure, a journey of discovery.

Like any journey, this one requires a certain amount of courage at the outset. Courage to do new things, think in new ways, entertain new ideas, some of which may surprise and startle you. Like any journey, too, this one requires at the outset a certain amount of confidence and a sense of excitement. Confidence in the guide and in the value of the goal. Excitement at the prospect of setting forth into unfamiliar territory, of testing your own ability to grasp new concepts and accept new points of view, some of which may seem not only unfamiliar but unorthodox.

However, I promise you that like any adventure undertaken with courage, confidence, and excitement, this one will reward you richly from beginning to end, every step of the way.

3

Before we start, you should know who I am, since I am to be your guide on this journey. I am a doctor, not of medicine but of natural science. I have taken my inspiration from the teachings of Hippocrates, Paracelsus, Father Kneipp, Hindhede, Bircher-Benner and other great teachers of ancient, medieval and modern times. The word doctor comes originally from the word "docere" meaning "to teach." Even if I were not licensed to practice a healing art, I would feel that I had earned the right to this title.

My friends and students have included some of the most famous, the most fabulous, and the most fortunate men and women in the world, as well as thousands upon thousands of average citizens. Rich and poor, celebrated and obscure, overnourished and undernourished, all these people had one thing in common.

They were hungry.

They were not hungry for more food, but for more life. For better health, younger bodies, keener minds. Because I have been able to satisfy their hunger, because I have taught them the secret of eating for health, good looks and greater vitality, these people, numbering hundreds of thousands, are my devoted friends and enthusiastically come to my lectures and classes in every large city in America and England.

I have three special qualifications for teaching people how to live longer. One is my own great relish for living. There was a time, many years ago, when I had a supposedly incurable disease and hope for me was given up. Perhaps I relish life more because at that time I had to fight for it. At any rate, I find it very good and very satisfying to be alive. Each year in May I celebrate my birthday; I like to receive the good wishes of my friends and the good thoughts of my students. But I refuse to get older. I celebrate each birthday not just as the end of another good and satisfying year of life but as the beginning of a new year of exciting work, travel and accomplishment.

My second qualification for teaching people how to live longer is my great relish for people. Perhaps the fact that I grew up in a large family (I am the eleventh of twelve children) has something to do with this.

As a dietitian, nutritionist, lecturer and writer, I travel constantly, all over the United States and Europe. Wherever I go, I meet more and more people. Many of these are People—spelled with a capital P. Many of these are my good friends. They include royalty, society leaders, stage and screen stars, statesmen, business executives, sportsmen, writers, philosophers, doctors, artists, scientists, teachers, preachers and—yes—a Civil War veteran.

I meet people in large and small cities, on trains, ocean liners and air liners. I meet them at Hollywood parties, in drawing rooms in New York, London, Paris and Rome. I meet them in the learned circles of Vienna and Copenhagen and in the crowds that gather around my lecture platform all the way from Boston, Massachusetts, to Seattle, Washington.

Also, I meet people in another place—on the shelves of the nearest library, wherever I happen to be—for my appetite for reading books by and about people is almost as great as my appetite for knowing them. Many of these library-shelf people also are People. Many of these, also, are my good friends.

My third qualification for teaching people how to live longer is my own great relish for longevity. I have always devoured everything bearing upon the subject of longevity—in the fields of nutrition, medicine, endocrinology, surgery, biology, bio-chemistry, psychiatry, philosophy, physical culture—wherever I could find it.

I have visited many of the famous watering places in Europe and the United States, and tested their special diets and regimes. I have visited doctors in their offices and sanatoriums, research scientists in their laboratories, and physical culturists at their health resorts and beauty farms. I have assembled rooms full of books and filing cabinets full of pamphlets, reprints and clip-pings dealing with my favorite subject. I have inquired into and experimented with or speculated upon everything I could find that anyone has said, thought, written, discovered, developed, invented, promised, prophesied or dreamed of, that had to do with the prolongation of life.

Why?

Well, I myself would like to live for a long time. I would like to live for at least one hundred years.

Would you?

I know what you are thinking. You are thinking, "This man is mad. Suppose I can live to be one hundred. Who wants to hang onto life—frail, dried-up, useless—just for the sake of prov-ing that it can be done?"

Who, indeed? Not I. You are thinking in old terms. I have told you that this book is an adventure into new ways of think-ing.

Do you want to live one hundred years if, at the age of one hundred:

Your body will not be wracked with aches and pains?

Your face will not look like a dried-up apple?

You can still be of definite use in the world?

Then come along with me.

In this book, this journey that we are taking together, I will teach you how to eat not merely to satisfy hunger, but to eat for health, good looks, youth, vitality, the joy of living. I will show you that you are not old at forty, fifty, sixty, seventy. That you need not be old at eighty, ninety—shall I go on?

Certainly I shall. I have friends and students who have passed seventy, eighty, ninety, and one hundred without getting old. I shall talk about them in this book. You will meet some of them and share their secrets.

You will learn how to nourish your entire body. You will learn how to eat so that your own blood stream will contain all the vital elements for nourishing the inside of your body, your arteries, glands, colon, bones, connective tissues. So that, whatever your age, you will *feel* young.

You will learn how to eat, also, so that your own blood stream will contain all the vital elements for nourishing the outside of your body, your muscles, skin, hair, teeth, eyes, complexion. So that, whatever your age, you will *look* young.

And you will learn how to eat so that your own blood stream will contain all the vital elements for full, energetic enjoyment of living, for nourishing your mind, heart, spirit, your total personality. So that, whatever your age, you will *be* young.

Forget your age. It does not matter. This is what matters: are you alive? Do you want to stay alive until you are one hundred or more years old? Do you consider the possibility that you may live to be one hundred an exciting idea? A challenge? An opportunity? A great adventure?

Then come along with me.

One moment more, before we start. What mental baggage are

you carrying? Some of it is excess baggage, I think. Let us discard that right now. Let us discard three pieces of mental excess baggage in particular.

The first one weighs ten tons. Here it is. Look your last at it before we throw it away.

"The days of our years are threescore years and ten."

Everybody "knows" that is true. Insurance companies have been founded on it. Retirement planners, pension planners, doctors, clergymen, you and you and your fathers and grandfathers before you, all "know" that the days of your years are threescore years and ten—seventy years. How do you know? Because you have read it in the Bible.

I, myself, know that it is *not* true. Facts and figures on longevity are a part of my lifelong study of the subject. Therefore I know that medical science, hand in hand with the science of nutrition, has been steadily increasing our life expectancy. Our potential life span, today, is longer than our parents thought possible. In the past twenty-five years the average life expectancy has been doubled. Today there are five million men and women in the United States who are over seventy. Twenty-five years from now that number will be doubled.

Definitely, the days of our years are *not* just the Biblical "threescore years and ten." I have grown impatient at hearing the phrase repeated. Recently I consulted the Bible to find out who was responsible for it.

I found it in the Ninetieth Psalm. Moses said it, in a lament to Jehovah. A lament, not a prophecy. It would surprise Moses, I think, to know that throughout the centuries his lament has been accepted as prophecy. He, himself, did not so accept it. He lived to be one hundred and twenty years old, and I was pleased to find, in another part of the Bible, that at the end of his life "his eye was not dim nor his natural force abated."

Now for the second piece of excess baggage. This one is not only heavy; it has sharp corners that prod painfully, reminding you to hurry, hurry, hurry. . . .

"It is later than you think."

Who said that? Inquiring, I found that it is an old Chinese proverb. What does it mean? No one could tell me. Later for whom? For the Chinese? Perhaps. In the Far East, millions of people live in ignorance of the simplest rules for health and hygiene. A few live to great age, due to unusual climatic and dietary conditions. The oldsters are so rare that pilgrimages are made and scientific expeditions organized to discover their special secrets. The average life span in the Far East today is about twenty-five years.

It is not later than *you* think. Thanks to the science of geriatrics, which is becoming increasingly interested in studying ways and means, not just of prolonging life, but of defeating the diseases of old age, you have plenty of time. Stop hurrying and getting panicky under the pricks of a meaningless Chinese proverb, or of any other proverb, including this one:

"Opportunity knocks but once."

That is excess baggage. Throw it away. Go to the biography shelves of your library. Find out how many men and women outstanding enough to rate a biography were Johnny-on-the-spot for that one knock of opportunity.

You will find the contrary to be true. You will find that it is not always seizing opportunity that is important. Far oftener, it is the sting of having missed opportunities in their youth that spurs mature men on to get things done. You will find endless examples of famous people who did their best work long after what you think of as middle age. Michelangelo, Goethe, Rembrandt, Victor Hugo, Titian, Emmanuel Kant, Rabelais, Benjamin Franklin—shall I go on? I could, indefinitely.

Opportunity keeps on knocking and its doors are everywhere. You are opening one door right now, as you read this book. A door to new health, new youthfulness, new and adventurous living.

Are you ready to start? One more discard. Let us discard that tiresome old portmanteau full of such standard phrases as "grow old gracefully," "act your age," and the like.

You are not growing old, gracefully, or any other way. As for acting your age, you are not concerned with your age. It is your youth that interests you.

Forget your age. It does not matter. This is what matters: Are you alive? Do you want to stay alive as long as you live? Not just living, but *alive*?

Then come along with me.

II. FORGET YOUR AGE

NOW, put this book down for a moment. Say to your-self, "I—this person sitting here in this chair—I can live to be one hundred years old." Say it aloud. Listen to your words. Repeat them.

This idea is new to you. It is a new kind of thinking. Take your time with it. Accept the idea of living to be one hundred. In imagination, extend your life forward, far into the future. Figure out what the calendar year will be when you are one hundred. Think what the world will probably be like, what new, interesting, unheard-of things probably will be happening. Say to yourself, "I shall be alive then. I can be alive in the year ——."

Accept those years. They are yours. This is not wishful thinking or idle daydreaming. It is simple acceptance of scientific fact. Science has increased your life span beyond your wildest expectations.

You can live one hundred years. This means that whatever your present age is, you are young.

Suppose you are forty-five. Heretofore you have been saying to yourself, "I am *forty-five*."

But now that you have been told that you will live to be one hundred, you are saying to yourself, "I am *only* forty-five."

What happens?

You begin to feel young!

It is an established scientific fact that all living creatures can live seven to fourteen times as long as the time required to attain maturity. Man attains maturity at the age of twenty; therefore he should live one hundred and forty years. Said the Russian Dr. Alexander A. Bogomolets: "A man of sixty or seventy is still young. He has lived only half his natural life. Old age can be treated just as any other illness because what we are accustomed to regard as normal old age is actually an abnormal, premature phenomenon."

Scientists have proved that life can be prolonged indefinitely. The Russian professor Kuliabko removed a human heart from a soldier killed in battle, and restored its action twenty-four hours after it had ceased beating. Another scientist, Briukhonenko, restored life in dead dogs by artificially renewing their blood circulation. *The stuff of which we are made is potentially immortal.* Many scientists have proved this, notably Dr. Alexis Carrel who experimented with a piece of heart tissue cut from a chicken and put into an ideal nutritive medium. This piece of chicken heart lived indefinitely, as long (and here is the important point for our Look Younger, Live Longer program) as the "broth" in which the tissue lived contained all the necessary nutrients, and as long as wastes were eliminated.

But to live long without growing old—how can that be done? From the dawn of recorded history, mankind has sought the fountain of youth.

You are as young as your glands, some scientists have said. The French scientist, Charles Edouard Brown-Séquard, believed that the secret of youthfulness lay in intravenous injections of extracts of animal testicles. Steinach, in Vienna, hoped that tying off the spermatic cord would flood an aging man's entire body with sex hormones and make him forget the calendar. Voronoff, in Paris, transplanted the sex glands of monkeys into male and female patients in the quest for rejuvenation. Following the same quest, American biochemists harked back to Brown-Séquard and developed testosterone, which has helped some and disappointed many.

You are as young as your colon, other scientists have said, notably the bacteriologist Metchnikoff. He believed that the body is prematurely aged by toxic bacilli released by the decomposition of food in the bowels. His secret of youthfulness was to wage war on toxic bacilli in the colon by marshaling against them armies of the beneficient bacilli contained in acidophilus milk and yogurt.

Said the English Dr. William Osler: You are as young as your arteries.

Said Bogomolets: You are as young as your connective tissues. Bogomolets made world-wide headlines by perfecting A.C.S. (antireticular cytotoxic serum) and stating that with regular injections of A.C.S., plus reasonable care, we can all live to be one hundred and forty.

Says the French Dr. Saint-Pierre in his book *Prolonger La Vie:* You are as young as your blood. In Paris today, people in search of rejuvenation are flocking to Dr. Saint-Pierre who, out of fresh young human blood, makes a serum and injects it into the bodies of aging men and women.

I believe that the answer lies not just in the glands, the colon, the arteries, the connective tissues, the blood, or in any *one* part of the body, but in the whole body.

Steinach himself realized that. He once said to me, "I have opened *one* door to the palace of truth. No doubt there are a hundred corridors I have overlooked, a hundred doors that others luckier than I will enter."

I believe that I am one of those lucky ones.

I believe that you are as young as you *look, feel, think, hope, believe and act*. And I believe that the way you look, feel, think, hope, believe and act depends on three things:

> Good food
> A strong, vibrant body
> An adventurous spirit

In short, I believe that *you are as young as your diet*.

The world over, scientists studying the extension of life are finding more and more evidence that the fountain of youth is *good nutrition*. Dr. Henry C. Sherman of Columbia University is considered one of the world's outstanding authorities on nutrition. In a lecture given before the New York Academy of Medicine, Dr. Sherman stated that, given the right selection of foods, human life can be greatly extended. Furthermore, says Dr. Sherman, the later years can be lived in much fuller measure of usefulness.

What is meant by good nutrition? First, it is adequate nutrition, giving the individual cells of the body not only the quantity but also the quality of nourishment they require. Second, it is balanced nutrition, supplying the body cells with vital nutrients in the proper proportion. Scientists are unanimous in agreeing that overnutrition, through excess calories stored as fat, can contribute materially to physical deterioration and the aging process.

As a simplified, perhaps crude, illustration, think of your body as a motor car. It is made of protein, inside and out. Arteries, glands, colon, connective tissue; muscles, skin, bones, hair, teeth, eyes: all contain protein and are maintained and rebuilt with protein. Fats and carbohydrates are your body's oil and gasoline; they are burned together to produce energy. Vitamins and minerals are its spark plugs, essential to the utilization of food and its assimilation into the blood stream.

It is a marvelously sturdy motor car, this body of yours—marvelous in its ability to maintain and rebuild itself. Given care, consideration and respect, it will function smoothly, on and on. Provided that none of its important organs have been allowed to break down, it can and will heal and regenerate itself at any age. It cannot be neglected or abused. It must be fed and cared for faithfully. When it does not hit on all cylinders, it must be examined by an expert mechanic who can not only find out what is wrong but detect hidden weaknesses, forestall serious breakdowns. Even when it is functioning adequately it should have regular over-all check ups, preferably always at the same "machine shop" where its history is known and its special characteristics and needs are understood.

Headed by the Mayo Brothers in Rochester, Minnesota, and Johns Hopkins Hospital in Baltimore, Maryland, human "machine shops" are springing up all over America. Wonderful clinics staffed with top-notch physicians, equipped with the most superb diagnostic facilities in the world, equipment which private doctors could not possibly afford. Doctors at such clinics look for specific symptoms, but more than that, they consider the individual as a whole—his body, his mind, his special circumstances and problems. They are interested, these expert "body mechanics," in the over-all picture. Their aim is to arrest deterioration and more, to forestall such deterioration, prevent it.

One by one, the so-called infectious diseases of old age are being controlled. Diabetes gives way to insulin and diet. Heart disease, hardening of the arteries, arthritis, strokes, high blood pressure—all are giving ground to science. I am convinced that with our growing knowledge of prevention, plus the immense progress the science of nutrition is making, America is leading he world into a new era, a Look Younger, Live Longer Era.

III. THE IDEAL DIET FOR LONG LIFE

*A*GE IS a physiological and psychological matter; it has no relation to the calendar. Examination of men and women over one hundred years of age at some of our famous clinics revealed that they had four outstanding qualities:

Strong digestive juices

A slow, rhythmic heartbeat

Good elimination

Happy dispositions

Let me introduce to you one of the happiest people I know. I first met her seven years ago. She had worked with Wallace Beery, Sonya Henie, Charles Laughton, Don Ameche, Bette Davis, James Stewart and a dozen others, but I did not know that. To me she was one of the hundreds of people who had crowded into a large auditorium in Los Angeles to hear me lecture.

I had never seen her before but I recognized her at once. She was one of my People. I knew by the way she sat—erect and disciplined, her shining white head resting proudly on straight shoulders. I knew by her face—strong as well as sweet, revealing inner beauty as well as beauty of line and feature.

She was a Person, no question about it. After my lecture, I saw her among the crowd gathering around the platform to meet me. We shook hands, and then I realized that she was an actress, too.

"Tell me," she said, her eyes sparkling with humor, her trained, resonant voice carrying clearly. In mock despair she put her hands on her stomach, which was perhaps not quite as flat as it might have been. "Tell me—*what* am I going to do about this *jelly belly?*"

Of course she brought the house down. That was seven years ago. Adeline de Walt Reynolds was then eighty-two.

At the age of sixty-five, she told me, having raised four children and helped raise a raft of grandchildren, she had decided to go to college. At sixty-nine, she was graduated from the University of California. Then Hollywood discovered her and the new star "Grandma Reynolds" was born. At the age of eighty-two, with thirteen years of stardom behind her, she saw no limit to the years of stardom ahead of her. *If* she could get rid of her "jelly belly."

That was not difficult. With a lifelong habit of regular exercise, a natural talent for relaxation, and the drive that comes from sheer zest for living, she had long since made of her body a well-trained, responsive instrument. Her basic dietary habits already were excellent; I advised only such changes as would make sure that her diet contained many, many of the good proteins needed to rebuild tissue more firmly and strengthen the natural "muscular corset" which has been given to all of us to protect the abdomen, the most vital and vulnerable region of the body. I added brewers' yeast to her diet and taught her the one setting-up exercise which I consider indispensable—the Stomach Lift. She bought herself two Body Slant boards—one a plain board, the other with a motor attached which mildly rocked her to sleep after a hard day's work at the studio. (I shall have more to say about the Stomach Lift and about Body Slant boards later.)

Six months passed. I lectured again in Los Angeles. Again Grandma Reynolds was in the audience. She was at my elbow the minute my lecture was over.

Her head was prouder than ever; her eyes were full of excitement and delight. She had just begun work on a new picture, she told me. It was the best role she had had yet. She was starring with Bing Crosby in "Going My Way."

The "jelly belly"?

Neither of us even mentioned it. Grandma Reynolds was as flat across the midriff as I am.

Nowadays, Grandma Reynolds is a television star in a charming program in which she tells modern bedtime stories to youngsters. What is her secret for long life, good health and happiness? She herself could not tell you. She could tell you that she has a strong constitution, that she has always loved life and believed in living each day to the full. She does not know her own secret. She has never analyzed it. Her secret is that all of her life she has followed *instinctively* the basic principles of the Look Younger, Live Longer program.

Long ago I discovered that my friends and students who are youthful at seventy, eighty and ninety had many of the same principles and beliefs that I had. The difference was that, while I had arrived at my principles and beliefs through study, research and experiment, they had arrived at theirs intuitively. It had been their lifelong habit to eat a balanced diet, keep their bodies in top-notch condition and maintain a cheerful, positive attitude of mind. I found that they knew without being told that it is better to undereat than to overeat, that they had been given, apparently by the good fairies who presided over their cradles, a supreme gift—the gift for complete body relaxation.

I have checked this evidence over and over again. Another outstanding example of its soundness is a good friend of mine who is now 103 years old—Hiram R. Gale, a veteran of the Civil War.

I met him more than ten years ago. In full uniform, complete with medals and decorations, this grand old soldier stood long in line at the reception which followed a lecture I gave in Seattle, Washington. He was erect, buoyant, with bright blue eyes and rosy skin.

"I wanted to shake your hand," he said. "I listened to every word you said. Not that I needed telling. Been doing everything you talk about as far back as I can remember."

A "natural" Hauser student all his life, Hiram Gale has, for the past eighteen years, since he went to Seattle to live with his son and daughter-in-law, been a literal follower of my regime. His daughter-in-law has taken every Hauser course given in Seattle since 1932. A real student, she studies, knows and practices Hauser teachings and as a result, Hiram Gale, at the age of 103, is exceptionally healthy, happy and ambitious. His big ambition—to be Commander-in-Chief of the G.A.R.—was fulfilled in 1945–46. Now it is his great ambition to be the Civil War veteran to outlive all Civil War veterans—an ambition which bids fair to be realized, for there are fewer than twenty veterans still alive and I feel sure that in body, mind and spirit Hiram Gale must be the "youngest" of them all. All Seattle knows and honors him; hopes that his greatest wish comes true.

In following my program, you are doing *consciously* what such a person has, for most of his life, being doing unconsciously. You are far more fortunate than he has been. All he had to rely on was superb physique and naturally sound instincts; you have the whole new and ever-developing science of nutrition at your service. With its help, even without superior physique, you can not only match him and others like him, in agelessness, but surpass them.

What you eat between the ages of 40 and 60 determines how you feel, look and think at 70 and 80. Now is the time to take stock of yourself. Now is the time to discard myths of "age," and concentrate on agelessness. Now is the time to discard careless habits and swing into the Look Younger, Live Longer way of life. *Health can be rebuilt at any age. Well and wisely fed, the body and all its organs are capable of reaching 100 or more without any vital part wearing out. There is no reason why YOU cannot attain 70 or 80 as free from physical ills as you were at 30.*

ENJOY YOUR FOOD

It was stated recently in one of the medical journals that 75 percent of the senior half of our population suffers from malnutrition. Studies reveal that most people over sixty suffer from six to eight nutritional deficiencies. My own personal observation corroborates these facts; rarely do I find, among the thousands of people—rich and poor—who come to me for advice, a person midway in life who does not show some symptoms of malnutrition.

Many things may contribute to this needless "running down" of life. With years of food for food's sake, the appetite becomes dull. With lessening of appetite, interest in preparing and eating good foods lessens. Perhaps mealtime is lonely. Loss of teeth may make chewing difficult; one may consider eating a tedious task to be finished as quickly and easily as possible, without thought of its life-giving potential.

Food is made for man. By all means, let us enjoy it. I believe in eating all kinds of good food, either fresh or properly cooked (never overcooked) in infinite variety. I believe in heightening the flavor of meats and sauces with herbs and mild spices, much as the French people do. I hope to see the day when everyone will not only consider a large, crisp salad as an important part of the main meal but will eat it *as the first course of the meal, when appetite is keenest.* Fruit should become the favorite dessert, either fresh or stewed in the modern manner with honey. (See Lady Mendl's *compote des fruits* on page 282).

Every mouthful you eat either does you good or harm. The secret of agelessness, after forty, lies in eating intelligently, in *liking* to eat only those foods which are good for you. This becomes easy, as you learn about food values, learn the values also of vitamins and minerals. It becomes exciting to feel yourself a kitchen chemist rather than a kitchen slave.

VITAMINS AND MINERALS

Protein keeps your body in repair, keeps it firm, keeps it functioning. Carbohydrates and fats keep you active, full of energy.

Vitamins are your body's best friends. They have many functions. Here are some which should interest you most:

Vitamin A is the "glamour" vitamin, helps produce smooth skin, bright eyes; helps build up resistance to infections and diseases. The vitamins of the ever-growing B family help to stabilize your heart, your nerves, and are vital for normal elimination. Vitamin C helps to keep all parts of your body young and pliant. Vitamin D assists in keeping teeth and bones strong, straight and firm; it also helps you to relax because it aids the body in using calcium efficiently. Vitamin E, the most hotly debated of all vitamins, helps to ward off many "old age" diseases.

Your body needs many minerals to prolong youth and zest for

life. Minerals help maintain water in the body, influence gland secretion, keep blood and tissue fluid from becoming either too acid or too alkaline. Calcium and phosphorus give hardness to teeth and bones. Older people need calcium and more calcium. Calcium (plus vitamin D) stabilizes the nerves, brings calmness, relaxation, sound sleep. Iron regulates the progress of oxygen and carbon dioxide in the blood stream, that "river of life" which the French Dr. Sainte-Pierre declares to be the fountain of youth. Iodine aids the thyroid gland to produce thyroxin, which maintains your urge for work and play, and prevents the body from putting on "middle-aged fat."

I believe that the ideal diet for long life is plenty of protein (milk, especially yogurt; eggs, lean meat, lean fish, fresh cheese), plenty of fresh green and yellow vegetables, vegetable juices, fruit, fruit juices and 100 percent whole grain cereals and flour. I believe, also, that everyone over forty should supplement his diet with optimum, not minimum, daily requirements of vitamins and minerals. *Do not try to substitute vitamin pills for food vitamins.* Without a sound basic diet, vitamin and mineral pills can do you no good.

Merely by adding generous amounts of such essential nutrients as calcium foods and vitamin A foods, the span of life can be lengthened. Studies also have shown that the life span can be prematurely *shortened* by inadequate diet, by lack of essential nutrients such as the important amino acids found in good proteins. The studies made by Dr. T. S. Gardner are an exciting example of the fact that you are as young as your diet. Using normal, healthy animals in his studies, Dr. Gardner gave additional amounts of vitamin B6 (pyridoxin) to one group. Their life span was increased by 10.5 percent. For a similar group, yeast nucleic acid was added to the diet, and their life span thereby increased by 11.3 percent. A third group of animals achieved a life-span increase of 27.8 percent when their diet was supplemented with pantothenic acid. Spurred by these surprising results, Dr. Gardner added all three—pyridoxin, yeast nucleic acid and pantothenic acid—to the animals' diet and made the amazing discovery that the life span was *increased 46.6 percent;* nearly half again as long as had formerly been thought possible. (Brewers' yeast contains all three of the above food factors.)

Proteins and more proteins. B vitamins and more B vitamins. According to Dr. Henry C. Sherman, whose findings I have seen consistently corroborated throughout my many years of active service in the nutrition field, first class proteins plus the complete family of B vitamins are indispensable for long life with the retention of the characteristics of youth.

THE WONDER FOODS
(VITAMIN B AND ITS FAMILY)

Get acquainted with, and *use every day for the rest of your long life,* these five wonder foods: powdered brewers' yeast (available plain or flavored), powdered skim milk, yogurt, wheat germ, and blackstrap molasses. *Any one of these five foods, used daily, can probably add five youthful years to your life.*

BREWERS' YEAST

This wonder food has been found to contain 17 vitamins, including the entire B family; 16 amino acids and 14 essential minerals. It contains 46 percent protein, yet is almost zero in sugar, starch and fat.

Powdered brewers' yeast can be added to milk, water, tomato juice, grapefruit, pineapple and other fruit juices. To mix the yeast, pour a pint of liquid into a quart jar, add 4 heaping tablespoonfuls of the yeast and stir moderately; then finish filling the jar with liquid and place it in the refrigerator. As the dissolved yeast will settle to the bottom of the jar, it should be stirred again each time you pour a glassful.

If you do not care for the taste of plain powdered brewers' yeast, it may be purchased in flavored form. I, myself, enjoy a celery-flavored yeast mixed with unsweetened pineapple juice. (See Look Younger recipe on page 264.)

Brewers' yeast, powdered skim milk, yogurt, wheat germ and blackstrap molasses can all be purchased at health food stores. None of these foods, except yogurt, need be kept in the refrigerator.

POWDERED SKIM MILK

The value of powdered skim milk lies in its richness of fat-free protein, calcium, vitamin B_2 (riboflavin) and other nutrients. I do not suggest that it be substituted for fresh milk, but that it be used in every possible way to fortify other foods. By beating half a cup of powdered skim milk into a quart of fresh milk, you obtain the value of 2 quarts of milk in the volume of 1 quart.

Fresh milk fortified with powdered skim milk has added richness and flavor, both as a beverage and for use in cooking. A half cup or more of powdered skim milk can also be added to breads, waffles, muffins, cream sauces, soups, custards, junkets and the like without making other changes in the recipes.

Be sure to keep your powdered skim milk in air-tight containers (such as vacuum pack coffee tins) because it absorbs moisture so readily that, if left open, it can be ruined within an hour on rainy or foggy days. Kept dry, it will retain its fine flavor and powdery texture for years.

YOGURT

While excellent yogurt can be purchased in dairy and health food stores, the homemade variety is far less expensive and can, if made with powdered skim milk, be fortified with twice the amount of protein, vitamin B₂, calcium and other nutrients.

My favorite yogurt is made by beating into a pint of water the following ingredients: 1½ cups of powdered skim milk; 3 tablespoons of previously made (or commercial) yogurt; and 1 large can of evaporated milk. When this mixture is beaten smooth, it should be added to 1 quart of water and poured into glasses which are set in a large pan containing enough warm water to reach the top of the glasses. The pan should then be set over a warming unit, pilot light, or simmer burner and the temperature of the water kept between 105 and 125 degrees Fahrenheit.

If an even temperature cannot be maintained within this range of heat, it is worthwhile to buy a yogurt maker.

The yogurt should thicken and be ready to chill in 3 hours. If it requires longer time, the temperature probably has run too low.

Yogurt can be eaten plain; seasoned with chives or other herbs; served with fresh or canned fruits; or made into a sundae with maple syrup, honey or blackstrap molasses.

Yogurt is a "must" on the Live Longer diet. Among the Bulgarians, where yogurt is a part of each meal but where diet is not outstanding in other respects, the life span is longer than that of any other peoples in the world; Bulgarians are credited with retaining vigor and virility and the characteristics of youth to an extremely advanced age.

The last census taken before the war in Bulgaria showed that for each million inhabitants, 16 lived 100 years or more; whereas here in the United States only 9 in a million reach the century mark and these are not nearly as spry and young-looking as the Bulgarian centenarians.

Yogurt is also an excellent food for those who are ill, as the milk proteins are already partially digested by bacterial enzymes during the culturing process and the milk calcium has been dissolved in the lactic acid of the yogurt, making it easier to absorb. In the intestinal tract, the bacteria of yogurt help to keep in check the putrefactive and pathological organisms which cause discomfort and gas.

Probably most important of all, however, is the fact that yogurt bacteria apparently manufacture generous amounts of the B vitamins in your digestive tract, where they are readily absorbed and distributed throughout the body.

WHEAT GERM

This is one of the best sources of vitamin E, iron, and all B vitamins, and a half cup of it contains four times as much protein as is found in an egg.

Wheat germ may be cooked in milk as a cereal, or added to hot and cold cereals. Excellent hot cakes, waffles, muffins and breads can be prepared by substituting from one half to one cup of wheat germ for an equal amount of flour in the recipe.

If you own one of those electric blending gadgets, you can make delicious drinks with a pint of any fruit juice, a small section of banana, and half a cup of wheat germ.

BLACKSTRAP MOLASSES

This is not only an excellent source of many B vitamins, but also of iron, calcium and other minerals. Blackstrap molasses is a by-product of sugar refining and contains all of the minerals and heat-stable vitamins of the original cane juice. It may be eaten with a spoon, or stirred into milk, or used as a substitute for sugar and syrup.

FORTIFIED MILK

A drink guaranteed to increase the health of any person, regardless of age, is fortified milk. This is prepared by putting into a beater (electric mixer) the following ingredients: 1 pint of milk; 4 heaping tablespoons of brewers' yeast; 1 cup of powdered skim milk; 1 tablespoon or more of blackstrap molasses. When the mixture is beaten smooth, another pint of milk should be stirred into it. The result is a delicious drink which is amazingly rich in calcium, iron and all the B vitamins as well as protein value equal to seven large steaks. I recommend this drink especially as a between-meal beverage or before going to bed.

AMINO ACIDS

A word should be said about protein hydrolysates, or amino acids, which are now being widely advertised. Unfortunately, they are somewhat unpalatable and extremely expensive. Furthermore, as one of the essential amino acids, tryptophane, is sometimes destroyed in the preparation of protein hydrolysates, these cannot serve as a substitute for complete protein. When sugar is added to make them better tolerated, their composition is no better than powdered skim milk.

Instead of these expensive prepared amino acids, it might be far better to obtain adequate proteins from powdered skim milk, brewers' yeast, and wheat germ. If necessary to aid complete digestion, enzyme tablets could also be taken.

If the five wonder foods—brewers' yeast, powdered skim milk, yogurt, wheat germ and blackstrap molasses—become a part of your daily diet, you can be sure that essential proteins, all the B vitamins, calcium, iron and other minerals are amply supplied.

In addition, give consideration to obtaining the most dependable sources of vitamins A, C, D, and E.

VITAMIN A

Large amounts of yellow and green vegetables and fruits; liver, butter and milk; all are good sources of the potent vitamin A.

It may be that with the passing years you have eaten too-small amounts of these foods; digestion and absorption of nutrients may have become less efficient. If so, extra vitamins are necessary to rebuild good health. Sometimes salads and firm-textured vegetables are not completely digested even by very young persons and they are unquestionably difficult to eat with ill-fitting dentures or without teeth. If for any reason you are undernourished (and remember that when I urge everyone over forty to "undereat," I am most decidedly *not* suggesting that you allow yourself to become undernourished) or if teeth make chewing difficult, balance your diet and see your dentist without delay. In the meantime, supply existing vitamin A deficiencies by taking the vitamin in capsule form.

Vitamin A capsules are available in potencies of 25,000 to 50,000 units each. The amount needed will vary with the individual, but if the budget allows, it is desirable to take about 25,000 units daily.

VITAMIN C

The potent vitamin C apparently plays a very important part in the prolongation of youthful characteristics. One of its principal uses in the body is to maintain elasticity and strength of the connective tissues.

Dr. Walter Eddy, in his book *The Vitamins*, points out the similarity between senility and scurvy, the deficiency disease caused by lack of vitamin C. In scurvy the symptoms appear rapidly, producing wrinkling of the skin and loss of elasticity, rarefaction of the bones and changes in teeth, gums, blood vessels and joints very similar to senility. The writings of Dr. Bogomolets stress that if health of the connective tissues can be maintained aging is greatly retarded.

It may be that the requirements of vitamin C increase with the increasing years of life, and changes in the intestinal walls and blood vessels may prevent the vitamin from being absorbed as readily as in earlier years. It is well, if you wish to keep your connective tissues young, to take 100 milligrams of vitamin C with each meal. This amount can be supplied by such natural foods as 3 glasses of orange juice; 3 green peppers; half a head of cabbage; or in 3 tablets of 100 milligrams each.

VITAMIN D

This potent vitamin is not supplied by foods in quantities sufficient to maintain good health and few people past adolescence can spend enough time in the summer sunshine to allow vitamin D to be absorbed into the body through the skin. Moreover, the natural oils of the skin, essential to formation of vitamin D, are all too often scrubbed off with excessive soap and water.

If you cannot spend one hour in the sun each day, it is best to fortify your diet with 1000 units of vitamin D preferably in the form of a fish-liver oil capsule.

VITAMIN E

Wheat germ is an excellent source of the potent vitamin E or alpha tocopherol. Because this E vitamin has become so important in the prevention of asthma, diabetes, heart disease and perhaps cancer, it would be wise to take an additional 30-milligram capsule daily.

WHY BOTHER?

Students sometimes ask, "Why must we be everlastingly intelligent about diet? Our forefathers knew nothing of vitamins, minerals, amino acids and the rest. They ate without thought of balanced diet and food values and maintained a high degree of health. Why must we bother always to eat in what you call the modern manner?"

The answer is, You must eat in the modern manner because you live in the modern age.

Our pioneer forefathers maintained a high degree of health on a seemingly carelessly chosen diet. But *their* grains, fruits and vegetables were grown in naturally rich topsoil which often ran ten feet deep. *Their* foods contained, many times over, a much greater vitamin and mineral quota than ours and far greater quantities of complete protein. Also, their meat, eggs and milk were much richer in nutrient than ours because more nutritious food was available to their animals.

Our pioneering forefathers also spent many hours of each summer day out in the open and their bodies were able to store quantities of vitamin D for immediate and winter use. They did not know that the rays of the sun form vitamin D in the oils *on* the skin, which is then absorbed into the body; they simply acquired their quota in the course of normal living. These sturdy pioneers had little soap and no hot water heaters and so could not easily prevent the formation of vitamin D by scrubbing all the natural oils from their skin. Needless to say, I am in favor of soap and hot water; it must be recognized, however, that valuable natural vitamin D lost by frequent bathing must be replaced in our diet.

Fortunately also for our forefathers, they did not know how to refine and destroy their flour and cereals. They were free from the foodless temptations of refined white sugar, cola drinks, candy bars and elaborate bakery products which deteriorate health and invite old age.

If *you* could obtain foods grown from such soils as theirs, if you could duplicate their outdoor life and dietary frugality, you also might Look Younger, Live Longer without giving thought to nutrition. But who among us can do that? Our only choice is to select our foods wisely and to fortify them with the inexpensive "wonder foods" plus the best balanced vitamin formulas obtainable in capsules or tablets.

I advocate the use of whole grain flours and cereals instead of devitalized or so-called "enriched" varieties both for cooking and for the crusts of pies and pastries. I hope to see the day when natural sugar (blackstrap molasses, honey, maple syrup) will be used instead of devitalized white sugar, when cola drinks will be avoided as enemies to long life.

I hope to see the day when everyone (especially everyone over forty) will undereat, never overeat and will as a matter of course include in the daily diet brewers' yeast, yogurt (or milk or buttermilk) fortified with powdered skim milk, wheat germ and blackstrap molasses. I would like to see everyone over forty drink café au lait (half coffee, half milk) or, better still, if you are sensitive to the caffein and tannic acid of coffee and tea, I suggest a drink consisting of two teaspoons of blackstrap molasses stirred into one half cup of very hot water to which hot milk may be added. This tastes quite good and is extremely healthful.

I hope, also, to see the day when everyone over forty will, as a matter of course, be moderate about drinking and smoking. Drinking in moderation is not harmful. There is no objection to beer, if the waistline can stand it. Wine is alkaline and contains natural digestive enzymes; taken in moderation it aids digestion; European doctors recommend wine with dinner for this reason. Wine is festive and cheerful. I have always believed that there should be pleasure, above all, in eating. The argument against hard liquor is that it is high in calories and diminishes interest in good food. It is also acid-forming and creates the need for more and more vitamins, especially those of the B family.

In moderation, smoking is not harmful; after meals it can be relaxing. I find, however, that excessive smokers always eat badly and keep their bodies starved of necessary proteins, vitamins and minerals. This makes them jittery and feeling jittery, they reach for another cigarette.

Overcome the habit of excessive smoking, if you have it. This takes character and determination, but wise diet will help you. When the body is satisfied with plenty of good food, especially with large amounts of calcium foods (the great balancer), it is much easier to reduce smoking to the point where it is a pleasure and not a curse.

THE TIME IS NOW

Frequently I hear the wishful remark, "Maybe some day they'll find cures for degenerative diseases." Let us stop waiting for cures and practice prevention by applying to our own lives, RIGHT NOW, the wonderful discoveries of nutrition. Here are significant discoveries:

Heart disease, high blood pressure, diabetes, arteriosclerosis, and cancer have increased tremendously since grain was first milled and vitamin E and all the B vitamins discarded in the refining process. Breads and cereals formerly were the most dependable sources of these vitamins.

No vitamin E and only two of the sixteen or more known B vitamins are added to devitalized bread ironically publicized as "enriched." What strange mathematics—to take away sixteen and only add two, and call the result "enriched." Such misbranding should be dealt with under the Pure Food and Drug Act. White, bleached flour is void of all life-giving elements and should be plainly marked "devitalized," not "enriched."

In countries where the devitalizing of grain has been forbidden, as in Belgium during the First World War, deaths from heart disease, arteriosclerosis, diabetes, high blood pressure, and cancer were reduced within a year.

While the death rate in Belgium dropped among people of all ages during the time the devitalizing of flour was forbidden, the decrease was greatest among persons over sixty-five years of age. Such findings strongly indicate that some of the most serious degenerative diseases are of dietary origin.

There remains no doubt that heart disease, high blood pressure, and arteriosclerosis could be reduced, and the incidence of cancer and diabetes decreased, if nutrition were adequate and health were planned rather than left to haphazard chance.

How can we apply the scientific findings which promise us vigor and health throughout the years of life? The answer is amazingly simple. Apply the basic rules of the Live Longer diet. See to it that your daily menu furnishes ample amounts of all known nutrients—all vitamins, all minerals, proteins, fats, natural sugars and starches—and eat only unrefined foods which supply known nutrients as well as many nutrients not yet identified by our chemists.

IV. YOU CAN LIVE A HUNDRED YEARS

FINAL DIET FOR LONG LIFE   35

known nutrients, all vitamins, all minerals, proteins, fats, nat-

DEPEND ON YOUR HEART

ES, depend on your heart. It is one of the sturdiest and most resilient organs of your body. Heart disease is called Public Enemy Number One, but it is an enemy which you yourself can capture if you will. Much has been learned about heart criminology in recent years. With wise diet, medical guidance and confidence in your heart itself, you can give that excellent organ at least one hundred years of strong, buoyant life. Your heart wants you to live; it is telling you so. Listen calmly to its quiet, inner voice and give it the co-operation it asks for.

Eat intelligently, every day, every month, every year. Your heart wants vitamins, particularly B vitamins. As evidence of this, it has long been known that the B vitamins are required in much larger amounts by anyone doing strenuous physical work. Functional heart disease has been experimentally produced in human volunteers by Dr. Russell Wilder of the Mayo Foundation, and by Dr. Norman Jolliffe of Cornell University Medical School. In each case, the volunteers were given a diet adequate in all respects except for vitamin B1, or thiamin.

Within two or three days, bradycardia (or slow pulse) developed; soon tachycardia (rapid pulse) was experienced on exertion. As the condition became more severe, there was an alternating slow and rapid pulse with the rapid pulse soon gaining the upper hand. The heart became enlarged, and electrocardiagrams showed it to be abnormal.

The thiamin-deficient person quickly becomes aware of palpitation, or conscious of heart beats. Dr. Jolliffe used as his subjects hospital internes who were doing strenuous physical work. Their thiamin requirements were so high, because of their work, that heart abnormalities developed in only four days' time on a deficient diet.

Rapid pulse can also be produced whenever calcium is undersupplied. Calcium is necessary for relaxation of the muscle tissues, between heart beats, and vitamin D is needed to absorb calcium into the body efficiently.

A lack of vitamin E also appears to be an important factor in heart troubles. Within recent years, Dr. E. V. Shute and his associates in London, Ontario (Canada), found that persons suffering from almost any type of heart disease—thrombosis, coronary occlusion, angina pectoris, damage left by rheumatic fever, or other abnormalities—frequently made marked recoveries when vitamin E was added to the diet.

Shortness of breath, chest pains and other symptoms of heart disease have disappeared within two or three days after massive doses of vitamin E were given. Dr. Shutes and his associates have recommended that as much as 90 milligrams of vitamin E, or alpha tocopherol, be taken after each meal for a month. During the second month, 60 milligrams of E should be taken after each meal. Thereafter, 30 milligrams should be continued indefinitely.

One of my students, a sixty-three-year-old biology professor, had suffered from angina pectoris for eight years. Attacks were becoming more severe and more frequent, occurring as often as once a week, and sometimes daily. Shortly after Dr. Shute's work was published, a physician put my student on a program of massive doses of vitamin E. His relief was immediate and dramatic. That was nearly three years ago; he has suffered no major attacks since then. There have been but two or three minor flare-ups and these only under pressure of overwork.

While the action of vitamin E is not yet fully understood, it is known that muscle tissues, well supplied with vitamin E, require less oxygen than when the vitamin is lacking or inadeequate. A diet rich in vitamin E, therefore, is a sound protective measure against trouble from heart ailments in which the blood supply to the heart muscles is cut off by a clot and the oxygen supply is lessened temporarily.

If you would stay young in heart, follow the Live Longer diet. Get vitamin E daily, either by eating half a cup of wheat germ (its richest natural source) or by taking capsules of wheat germ oil. Make sure that the wheat germ oil has been extracted by the solvent method; ordinary cold press wheat germ oil does not contain all the needed factors. Be sure to obtain calcium in more than sufficient amounts. Get calcium in cottage cheese, milk and yogurt fortified with powdered skim milk, or in calcium tablets.

Be sure that your diet emphasizes—even overemphasizes—foods containing all vitamins of the B family. The B vitamins are soluble in water and hence cannot be stored in the body; they must be eaten every day. Get them from natural sources: from brewers' yeast, wheat germ, rice bran or polishings, blackstrap molasses and liver. Get them from yogurt, which contains bacteria capable of living in the intestinal tract and making B vitamins for you.

HARDENING OF THE ARTERIES (ARTERIOSCLEROSIS)

It must be understood that normal blood pressure varies constantly and can become unusually high during strenuous exercise, excitement or emotional stress. Only in cases where the blood pressure remains abnormally high, year after year, should hardening of the arteries be suspected. Even then it must be remembered that there are people who live long and happy lives in spite of arteriosclerosis.

This disease is caused by the formation of a hard, waxlike substance (cholesterol) in the walls of the arteries. Many arteries can become thus hardened before the blood pressure is affected, but eventually the thick deposits of cholesterol reduce the arteries to small, inadequate channels. Since the amount of blood in the circulatory system remains the same, the strain on the heart increases as the diameter of the plugged arteries decreases, and the blood pressure rises. You can illustrate this principle with a garden hose, by trying to force the same amount of water through a much smaller hose than would normally be used. Fatalities occur when the coronary arteries become completely plugged with cholesterol deposits.

Until the present time, little could be done to stop this hardening process. Doctors and patients alike said, "Advancing age causes it. It might as well be accepted gracefully." Nowadays, however, the picture is changing. I, myself, have seen hundreds of intelligent people put a halt to this process of hardening by following a low-fat diet, increasing their vitamin intake, and drinking freely of fresh green and yellow vegetable juices. I am delighted to report (and I believe that this fact alone would justify the publication of this book) that the experimental work of Dr. Lester Morrison and others has recently shown that the original cause of hardening of the arteries is dietary; the undersupply, probably over a period of many years, of three B vitamins in particular, cholin, betaine and inositol, appears to be the offending cause. These vitamins help the body use and transport fat and cholesterol.

Studies have also shown that when these B vitamins are generously supplied in the diet, arteriosclerosis is gradually corrected. The cholesterol deposits are apparently removed from the arterial walls and the blood pressure thus allowed to return to normal. This procedure requires from several months to a year or more, so be patient; remember that high blood pressure can correct itself when the arteries again are free from these waxy deposits and can again function normally.

Cholin, betaine and inositol are found, together with other sources of the B vitamins, in brewers' yeast, wheat germ, liver and whole grain breads and cereals. The richest source of cholin is brains; of inositol, blackstrap molasses. To stay young in heart, see that your diet contains all these natural sources of the B vitamins and, if you like them, eat calf or lamb brains once a week for extra amounts of cholin.

HEART TROUBLE AND DIET

It is my prediction that unless people learn to select their foods wisely, arteriosclerosis and high blood pressure will even increase. Why? Because they are not getting the *complete* family of B vitamins. There are many vitamins in the B family and their action is synergistic; that is, they work together. Increasing the intake of one or several B vitamins increases the need for all other vitamins of the B group.

Thousands of people are now taking tablets or capsules which furnish generous amounts of the cheaper B vitamins such as thiamin, riboflavin, niacin and pantothenic acid. Millions are eating bread "enriched" with thiamin and niacin. The need for the equally important and more expensive B vitamins such as betaine, cholin and inositol, as well as biotin, para-aminobenzoic acid, folic acid and others, is thus increased.

Therefore, I say, and it may seem a startling statement, that I suspect it will prove to be true that eating "enriched" bread and taking *incomplete* or single vitamin B tablets instead of the entire B complex family can result in increase of arteriosclerosis and high blood pressure. This alone is good and sufficient reason for taking your vitamins, whenever possible, in food form.

In cases where blood pressure is high, arteries hardened, or heart function abnormal, it is best to follow a low-fat diet as consistently as possible. The most important point to remember is to include in your diet the above foods rich in the B vitamins, especially cholin, betaine and inositol. These help the body to use fat and prevent harmful deposits of cholesterol from forming in the walls of the arteries. It has been found that when persons suffering even mild heart involvement caused by arteriosclerosis embarked on diet sprees high in fats but low in B vitamins, fatalities have occurred within as short a time as three months. A high-fat diet might have been recommended because of some other condition or because of the patient's desire to gain weight, and the B vitamins omitted through ignorance or negligence.

Animal fats such as butter, lard, suet, the fat found in eggs, meat, fish and poultry are all rich in cholesterol. It was first thought that only the cholesterol from these animal fats caused the increase in hardening of the arteries, but even vegetarians have been found to have excessive amounts of cholesterol, no doubt because their diet includes quantities of salad oils or fats in the form of mayonnaise, peanut butter, nuts or avocado, even though such fats are free from cholesterol. The body manufactures cholesterol from *any kind* of fat. Therefore, hold up your right hand and swear forever more to include in your diet optimum amounts of the B vitamins which prevent deposits of cholesterol from forming in the walls of the arteries.

If you are curious to know whether you have an excess of cholesterol in your blood, I suggest you let your doctor make a test; it is quite simple and inexpensive. This is one test which I hope the "human machine shops" of the future will make regularly.

Persons suffering from high blood pressure were formerly advised to avoid proteins. That idea has changed with recent research. A diet rich in protein can cause low blood pressure to increase to normal, but it cannot produce abnormally high blood pressure. On the contrary, protein intake should be more than adequate to keep the blood vessels strong. But since the proteins of eggs and cheese contain fats and cholesterol, the excellent fat-free proteins of brewers' yeast and powdered skim milk, cottage cheese, and lean meats should be heavily relied upon.

Salt also was formerly frowned upon, although it is needed daily to maintain normal health. Large amounts of salt can increase the blood pressure by holding excessive water in the body. Therefore, restriction of the use of salt is sometimes justified as a temporary measure when the blood pressure is dangerously high or in cases where the kidneys are so damaged that salt is not excreted.

Other good rules of diet should be observed when the blood pressure is abnormally high. Since vitamin C is necessary to maintain the strength and elasticity of normal blood vessels, this vitamin must be supplied in unusually large amounts, subject of course to your doctor's discretion.

Although the amount of liquid taken daily may not need to be restricted, not more than eight ounces should be drunk *at one time* if the blood pressure is hovering near the danger point. Taking several glasses of liquid at one time can easily increase the blood volume too rapidly. Digestion itself increases blood pressure, hence it is wise to divide the meals into six small ones rather than three large meals.

STOP THAT STROKE

Have you ever noticed that strokes and paralysis frequently occur on Thanksgiving Day or after New Year's celebrations when excitement, overeating and drinking all combine to increase an already too-high blood pressure? The body's blood vessels are a truly remarkable transport system through which the heart pumps several tons of blood each and every day. To keep these arteries strong, from the largest to the smallest, is an important task in our Look Younger, Live Longer program.

Naturally, all nutrients are necessary for this. But we have to thank the Hungarian Dr. Albert Szent-Gyorgyi for the discovery of vitamin P which helps to strengthen these important blood vessels that go to make up our river of life. To a friend who had weak blood vessels and who suffered from constant hemorrhages, Dr. Szent-Gyorgyi gave a crude extract made from fresh peppers (most plentiful in Hungary), lemons, oranges or grapefruit. The hemorrhages stopped promptly and Dr. Szent-Gyorgyi, who had received the Nobel Prize for the discovery of vitamin C, assumed that it was this vitamin which had strengthened his friend's weakened capillaries and stopped the hemorrhages.

However, when pure vitamin C was given, it did *not* stop hemorrhages, and this indicated that fruit and vegetable juices contain other factors which pure vitamin C does not contain. After much more research it was discovered that fresh green peppers and all citrus fruits contain other factors which pure vitamin C does not contain—a special factor which is strengthening to the blood vessels. This new factor was called vitamin P.

People whose skin bruises easily very often have weak capillaries and should by all means include both vitamin C and all of the vitamin P-containing foods in their diets. (See Live Longer recipes on page 257).

Here in America, Dr. James Couch discovered another blood-vessel-strengthening substance which promises to be a stroke preventative. This substance is called rutin and is extracted from green buckwheat. Smaller amounts are found in some flowers, in the leaves of elderberries, the stems of tomatoes and in barley. This rutin, which only your doctor should perscribe in concentrated form, has been of amazing help where blood vessels were dangerously weak and near the rupturing point.

Haphazard eating, constant tension and worry, can harm your blood vessels. Also there are a few drugs which can make blood vessels more fragile. These are aspirin, sulfa and stilbestrol which, therefore, should not be taken except on the doctor's advice.

In Sweden, Dr. G. F. Gothlin has made it part of his examination to test the strength or weakness of his patients' blood vessels. I hope that this simple test will also be applied in our "human machine shops" of the future so that by application of the Live Longer diet, use of vitamin P and rutin, patients can be helped to ward off hemorrhages and prevent strokes.

DIGESTIVE DISTURBANCES

You can be free from the digestive disturbances which often become increasingly frequent and distressing with the passing years. They are usually the result of inadequate diet. Their general cause is an undersupply of the B vitamins and of proteins in particular.

With insufficient B vitamins, not enough energy is produced and the contractions of stomach walls and intestinal tract, necessary for good digestion, slow down or cease. Consequently, food is not well mixed with the digestive juices and enzymes, and the semidigested food is not brought into proper contact with the absorbing surface of the intestinal wall where it can pass into the blood stream. Such undigested and unabsorbed food supports the life of millions of bacteria. Halitosis, flatulence, and distressing gas are the result.

A lack of adequate proteins can cause digestive abnormalities. The enzymes necessary to digest food are made of proteins containing all the essential amino acids. Where protein is inadequate or one or more of the essential amino acids is lacking, the digestive enzymes are insufficiently produced. Furthermore, without enough proteins, the tiny muscles surrounding the intestinal tract become as weak and stringy as old rubber bands; the normal movements of the intestinal tract cannot be maintained and still more undigested food serves to support bacterial growth.

Doctors at the famous Mayo Clinic have had the opportunity to study thousands of patients from every walk of life. They have discovered an important fact to which I invite the attention of all soda and alkalizer addicts. The fact is this: if a person's gastric juice is strongly acid, then he is likely to live longer. It has been found that acid secretion is normal when B vitamins are obtained in adequate amounts.

In our Look Younger, Live Longer program, we put forth every effort to preserve the natural gastric acidity of the stomach;

it prevents dangerous bacteria from getting into the intestinal tract. Never break down this first line of defense by taking alkalizers, soda and other neutralizers. *A strongly acid stomach is one of the requisites for a long and healthy life.*

If you have a nonacid or low-acid stomach, your doctor can give you a hydrochloric acid preparation to be taken before meals. If your digestion is normal, the pleasantest way of obtaining a necessary gastric acidity is to eat your salad first, especially if it is made with a tangy salad dressing which includes lemon, oil, vegetable salt, and some onions or garlic. Europeans have a glass of wine with their meals to aid digestion. Californians drink a glass of grapefruit juice as an appetizer. I suggest that you adopt any one of these simple procedures; they can compensate for a lack of free digestive acids and give you, besides, added vitamins and minerals.

The very small percentage of people who have a real excess of acid secretion (so-called hyperacidity) also should stop dosing themselves with soda and alkalizers; it does no real good. Instead, they should change their eating habits; a diet rich in proteins and optimum amounts of the B vitamins is needed. Equally important for these tense, high-strung persons (who often smoke to excess) is cultivation of the art of relaxation. They need to learn not only *what* but *how* to eat—with a serene mind, without noise, without aggravations.

You can also cause digestive problems by eating too rapidly, and under high nervous tension. Eating rapidly and carelessly causes quantities of air to be swallowed with the food. The air expands in the stomach as it heats to body temperature and may remain there to cause flatulence and gas pains, burping, belching and heartburn.

If ill-fitting dentures or too few teeth make thorough chewing impossible, then firm-textured fruits and vegetables should be mashed or puréed. Better still, their juices should be extracted and drunk through a straw, or made into cream soups.

Bear in mind that eating too rapidly, or with ill-fitting dentures or too few teeth to chew well, causes food to reach the stomach in pieces too large for the digestive enzymes to do their work effectively. By such procedures, you invite digestive troubles.

The obvious remedy for all self-invited digestive disturbances is, first of all, a sound nutritional diet adequate in all respects. Secondly, train yourself to eat slowly and chew thoroughly. Third, do not overload your stomach at one meal; have smaller and more frequent meals which can be readily digested by the few enzymes available.

To correct extreme cases of distress, these small meals should be made up of nonfibrous foods rich in proteins and B vitamins. Cream soups, milk drinks, custards or junkets made with fresh and powdered milk; wheat germ cooked in milk; brewers' yeast stirred into fruit juices; and broiled liver are recommended. Tablets containing digestive enzymes and a small amount of dried bile can be taken with each meal until your own digestive processes have been improved.

Follow the Live Longer Diet on Page 249 and thus avoid the lack of protein and B vitamins which causes so much digestive disturbance. Remember that sound digestion is the result of good health planning. It is an important step in our Live Longer program.

LAZY ELIMINATION

"A man whose bowels move regularly and normally will live very long," said Herodicus of Selymbria. That observation, made before the Christian era began, holds true to this day. Physicians have long noted that health and longevity are connected with the condition of the alimentary tract. Centenarians, who usually enjoy excellent digestion, can attribute a great deal of their longevity to the healthy functioning of the entire intestinal tract.

The most striking case of healthful longevity is that of Thomas Parr, a poor English peasant who worked hard until the age of 130, and died at the age of 152. Dr. William Harvey, the famous surgeon who discovered the circulation of the blood, personally performed an autopsy on Parr's body and was amazed at the findings. Even at 152, Parr's vital organs were in perfect condition; his heart was normal and the blood vessels unchanged; his testes were sound and normal, and until a few years before his death, he had enjoyed normal sexual relations.

In connection with Thomas Parr's astounding vitality, it is important to note that throughout his long life he had regular elimination. And note this: Parr was an *under*eater. His diet was largely made up of cheese, yogurt, many vegetables, and coarse dark bread made of whole grain wheat. He also enjoyed whey as a beverage (the calcium-rich water derived from sour milk). On a visit to London in the last year of his life, Parr began to eat many unfamiliar and heavy foods, and suffered accordingly. The change from good and simple foods to rich and overrefined foods, according to his biographer, rapidly undermined Parr's health and led to his death.

If digestive troubles and lazy elimination (constipation) have plagued you, begin now to adopt an adequate nutritional program and follow it daily for the rest of your long life. Constipation can exist only when energy production falls below normal. The *undernourished* muscles in the walls of the large intestine lose the power to contract sufficiently to effect a normal evacuation of body wastes, and lazy elimination is the result.

Ample supplies of the B vitamins aid the normal production of energy and almost any case of lazy elimination can be readily corrected by a diet rich in these vitamins. I recommend that half a cup of wheat germ, two or three tablespoons each of brewers' yeast and blackstrap molasses, and a pint of yogurt be taken daily until the stools become normally soft and readily eliminated. Blackstrap molasses has such excellent laxative qualities that some people will find a small quantity amply effective. On page 257 you will find appetizing recipes to aid you in making these wonder foods a part of your Live Longer program.

One purpose of the large intestine, or colon, is to retain water and allow it to be absorbed back into the blood stream. If food masses remain overlong in the colon, the wastes lose their water content and become hard and dry. Constipation, meaning a hard stool, is the result.

Dr. Martin Gumpert of New York has shown that chronic constipation, a national bad habit in the United States, can start severe disturbances of the whole digestive apparatus. Too many people become addicts of laxatives early in life, partly because of clever advertising and partly because of bad eating habits and laziness. Children are fed laxatives by intestine-minded mothers from the earliest age. Small wonder, then, that the natural function of bowel movement, which works like a clock *without artificial interference* and is well able to take care of its small disturbances, becomes degenerated in more and more adults.

Perhaps the most harmful method of correcting lazy elimination is by taking mineral oil or products containing it. Mineral oil is not digested. It readily absorbs the fat-soluble vitamins A,

D, E and K and washes them from the body with the feces. The *Journal of the American Medical Association* has repeatedly published warnings to physicians not to recommend mineral oil for human use.

The only laxative which I have recommended to my students all over the globe is a mixture of natural herbs. For correcting temporary constipation and for elderly people needing extra help, these chopped-up herbs have been most satisfactory. The formula that I use came originally from Switzerland. Since the war, excellent herbs are again being grown in the United States and this same Swiss formula is now being made up here. It can be obtained in health food stores throughout the nation.

In some rare cases where lazy elimination habits are of long duration, other special measures can be taken *temporarily*. A teaspoon of milk sugar stirred into a glass of yogurt or butter-milk can be taken three times daily. The laxative quality of milk sugar is caused by the fact that the action of bacteria in the large intestine transforms the grains of milk sugar into a gas which helps make the stools soft and bulky.

Or tablets of dried or dessicated bile can be taken temporarily with each meal. They are quite harmless *provided* that no strong cathartic has been added to them. When buying bile tablets, be sure to read the label and see that they contain no cascara and no phenolphthalein. As laxatives are always more or less irritating to the intestinal walls, they should *never be used habitually*.

In some extreme cases of lazy elimination, your physician may recommend a few internal irrigations, but these should only be given by experts. Habitual enemas can be harmful. They can cause the tiny muscles surrounding the rectum (like thousands of rubber bands) to expand so quickly that they break down, thus destroying the muscular strength.

The greatest harm done by lazy elimination is the mechanical injury (hemorrhoids) caused by irritation of the intestinal wall. When the diet is *kept adequate in all respects,* the stools are kept soft, hemorrhoids are prevented and any which may have formed usually disappear.

Where lazy elimination is due to muscular weakness and an enlarged, flabby belly, the diet must be made extra rich in good proteins and the B vitamins in order to re-establish good muscular tone. The Stomach Lift (*Bauchgymnastik*) as outlined on page 128 should be done habitually, on arising and before retiring, every day.

Commercial exploitation of the intestinal complex has been, and still is, quite ruthless. One need only study the advertisements in the subways, magazines and newspapers, to be convinced that constipation has indeed become a national bad habit. I agree with Dr. Gumpert that the addiction to laxatives should be stopped. Larger and larger doses become necessary as time goes on; thousands upon thousands of people find themselves struggling with the lazy elimination habit for the rest of their lives.

Overcoming chronic constipation begins with curing the addiction to laxatives. This may seem almost as difficult a job as curing a drug addict. Complete withdrawal of the daily dosage is the best, if most radical, way. After an unpleasant period of abstinence symptoms, the body usually finds its way back to a regular and spontaneous bowel movement. Regularity in habit, in sleeping, eating and elimination, is necessary if you would be free of intestinal worries. The lazy elimination habit has no place in our Live Longer program.

Bear in mind that in longevity tests, the spryest oldsters are always those who have maintained normal, natural daily elimination. At the St. Louis Clinic, among 200 men and women who had reached the fourscore mark, it was discovered that *all* had normal daily eliminations.

And while on the subject of better elimination, I would like to point out that the water closets in our elegant bathrooms belong to antiquity. Our plumbers and anatomists should get together to design a water closet which conforms to human needs. Nothing is so helpful to complete and easy bowel movement as the squatting position, and I see no reason why the water closet of the future cannot be designed and built so that the squatting position is automatically assumed.

Such a water closet need not be as unattractive as the old-fashioned contraptions in France and Japan (where you *must* squat whether you like to or not). I believe it could be simply and effectively designed to be lower at the back, thus permitting definite elevation of the knees. Until such time as that may be, many wise people have adopted the use of bathroom stools about ten inches high, on which to rest the feet during eliminations. This lifts the knees, bringing the thighs close to the abdominal muscles, and approximates the natural squatting position. I believe that the installation of properly designed water closets, anatomically correct, would be of immense help in banishing constipation, one of the great handicaps to our Live Longer program.

V. BUILD UP YOUR BODILY RESISTANCE

INFECTIONS

BY BUILDING up bodily resistance, you can reduce your susceptibility to many infections which are commonly accepted as inevitable in the second half of life.

Your blood stream is the river of life which can bring health and nourishment to every part of your body. This stream is a two-way river and (believe it or not) it is about 62,000 miles long. Flowing in one direction is your arterial blood stream which carries nourishment, together with the oxygen needed for its utilization, to the individual cells of your body. Flowing in the other direction is your venous blood stream which removes carbon dioxide and other waste matter from your body cells.

For the proper nourishment of every organ in your body and for building resistance to infection, the arterial blood stream must contain an adequate daily supply of nutrients. Protein is of first importance. Through the use of proteins containing all the essential amino acids, the body can produce its own army of antibodies and cells known as phagocytes which destroy bacteria and viruses invading your life stream. Experiments have shown that when a high protein diet replaces one low in protein, *as much as a hundred times more antibodies are produced within a week.*

As much as 80 to 100 grams of complete protein should be consumed daily, in order to build up good resistance to infections. At the beginning of an infection, the diet should consist largely of protein.

One of the cheapest, most palatable, most concentrated, and most completely digested of all protein foods is powdered skim milk. The addition of half a cup of dry skim milk to such dishes as cream soups, milk drinks, junkets, and custards will give you an unbelievable amount of protein value.

Peanut flour, which is 60 percent protein, is an inexpensive super-food that can be added generously to soups without altering their flavor. It is my conviction that high protein diets, including peanut flour and powdered skim milk, should be used liberally in all hospital diet kitchens. (See page 348 for high protein foods.) Remember that your body's life stream cannot be vitally healthy without the necessary amino acids contained in proteins.

Vitamins A and C are the two most important vitamins for building up resistance and combating infections. It is a well-known fact that epidemics are rampant during famines and wars when the diets are deficient in proteins and vitamins A and C. King and Menton have reported that resistance to diphtheria is increased by taking large amounts of vitamin C, and Kaiser reports that streptococci are less likely to be found in the tonsils of patients who have been given large amounts of this vitamin. Vitamin A is of particular value in combating infections of the lungs and bronchi; it maintains the health of the lining of the respiratory tract. As Dr. Walter Eddy has pointed out, "Vitamin A is necessary for resistance to germ invasions."

Vitamin A is found in all yellow and green vegetables and fruits, and in liver, cream and butter. It may not be possible to eat these foods in quantity during illness, in which case vitamin A requirements can be supplied by taking fish-liver oil capsules (of 25,000 or 50,000 units) immediately after meals. While the recommended quota of capsuled vitamin A will depend upon the severity of an infection, it usually ranges from 25,000 to 100,000 units daily through the convalescent period. In any case, massive doses are not harmful and any excess is stored for future protection.

For a list of other sources of vitamin A, see page 349. Make sure that your daily diet contains adequate supplies of this life-giving nutrient; it is "A" must for a healthy life stream.

Vitamin C, equally important to healthy resistance, is found in all fresh fruits and vegetables. Two or three glasses of fresh citrus juice daily will give you an adequate supply of the potent vitamin C so necessary to a smooth-flowing life stream. On page 354 you will find a list of other sources of vitamin C.

For those who cannot take that quantity of fresh juice daily, I recommend the substitution, when necessary, of a 100-milligram tablet of ascorbic acid with each meal.

One hundred milligrams of ascorbic acid (vitamin C) can be taken every two or three hours, to good advantage, at the beginning of any infection. Excellent results can be obtained, and healing speeded up in serious infections, by taking a *daily* amount of 500 milligrams of vitamin C (ascorbic acid) and 100,000 units of vitamin A, over a sixty-day period. I, myself, as well as thousands of my students, have warded off many troublesome infections by carrying out this vitamin A and C saturation method for sixty days before cold wintry weather sets in.

In combating any infection, the entire diet must be made adequate not only in large amounts of protein and the vitamins A

and C, but in all other nutrients as well. Exceptional requirements apply to a few specific infections.

Infections of the gall bladder or liver, such as hepatitis, require that fats be largely omitted from the diet, and that tablets
supplying the digestive enzymes and bile be taken with each
meal and mid-meal. Such tablets may be prescribed by your
doctor to eliminate the gas pains which are the most distressing
symptom of gall bladder and liver infections.

Infections of the kidney or bladder require that the urine be
made as acid as possible in order to combat the growth of bacteria. Fruits, fruit juices, and vegetables should be eaten sparingly. Citrus juices and blackstrap molasses (which furnish
unusually large amounts of alkaline minerals) should be avoided
until the urinary infection has been overcome.

In cases of urinary infection, the diet should consist of cooked
whole cereals, especially wheat germ, ground or broiled meats
and meat soups; milk, cheese and eggs.

In some infections, sulfa drugs are used as an emergency
measure to halt the spread of bacterial growth. It is a curious
fact that some harmful bacteria, once they have invaded the
body, thrive on the B vitamins. The sulfa drugs are effective because they destroy the B vitamins needed by the bacteria. That
is why exhaustion, skin rash, anemia, and other symptoms of
vitamin B deficiency follow the taking of sulfa drugs.

If an emergency arises and sulfa drugs are being used, all
foods rich in B vitamins should be temporarily avoided. However, when the infection has been cleared up and the drugs dis-
continued, *then* the diet should be made extremely rich in all
B vitamins to overcome the induced deficiency. For a speedy
recovery, add to your diet large quantities of brewers' yeast,

wheat germ, liver and blackstrap molasses. For other good sources of the B vitamins, see page 350.

Of particular interest to the man over forty is the avoidance of prostate gland infections. Among the primitive races of man, such infections are unknown, but here in America few men escape some prostate infection during the later years of life. If you will practice sound nutrition, infections of the prostate can be avoided. Experiments have shown that in laboratory animals, infections of the prostate gland are readily produced on a diet lacking sufficient protein and vitamins A and C.

Where prostate infections exist, the diet must be made more than adequate in all respects. Such a diet should include 100 grams or more of protein; 100,000 units of vitamin A; and 1,000 milligrams of vitamin C *daily* and should be continued through convalescence. (See special building diet on page 345.)

FOCAL INFECTIONS

No Look Younger, Live Longer program, be it ever so perfect and ever so perfectly followed, can succeed in its purpose if the food you put into your mouth is prevented from reaching the body organs for whose nourishment it is intended. And just as obviously, hidden or so-called "focal" infection must not be allowed to obstruct the free flow of venous blood and thereby lead to venous congestion.

The organs of your body can function properly and stay young and healthy *only* if the inflow of life-giving arterial blood and the outflow of waste-laden venous blood balance each other. Uninterrupted, *balanced* circulation is the basis of youth and health. When the circulation in any organ is thrown out of balance by a slowing up of the venous outflow, the cells of that organ do not get their proper amount of food and oxygen. Then they starve; their normal power to resist bacterial poisons and germs is weakened and the organs succumb to disease.

We who are traveling the road to long and vigorous life need to familiarize ourselves, as we go along, with a problem which has challenged and fascinated the medical profession ever since it was formulated 130 years ago—the subject of focal infection.

The focal infection theory has had its ups and downs, but it has never been completely discarded. Its failures have not proved that the theory was wrong, only that its practical application was often faulty. The main objection to the focal infection theory has always been that removal of a focus (usually teeth or tonsils) does not always cure the patient.

This is understandable when you realize that many tonsillectomies are incomplete and leave an infected tonsil stump which may be worse than the original tonsil. After such an operation, the stump becomes covered over by scar tissue which seals in the infection, forcing it to drain out into the blood stream.

Old-fashioned dentistry often is a source of focal infection, due in part to the antiquated practice of filling root canals in order to save teeth. Devitalized teeth, wherein the nerve has been extracted, become infected within a short time. Whether or not a tooth is still alive can easily be determined by a simple vitality test, should the X-ray show no sign of infection. Such hidden dental infections, draining into the blood stream, can cause arthritis and other serious diseases.

Anyone suffering from infected teeth and tonsils at the same time should by all means have the teeth troubles corrected first. The inflamed tonsils often will heal by themselves when dental infection has been removed. Infected tonsil stumps, however, cannot heal by themselves and always must be removed by an expert surgeon.

Dr. Otto Meyer of New York, specialist for arthritis and phlebitis, has been treating diseases of the veins for over a quarter of a century and experience has taught him that infections which defy other treatments can be overcome by restoring a normal balanced circulation in the affected organ.

According to Dr. Meyer, arthritis and apoplexy are two of the most common infections due to venous congestion. Glaucoma and other diseases of the eye; ear conditions (as persistent ringing of the ears and other noises); certain types of neuralgia, varicose veins, and neuritis (especially trifacial neuralgia and sciatica) are others.

Does it seem strange to you that so many apparently unrelated diseases could be due to the same cause? Not if you realize that the proper functioning of *every* organ depends on normal circulation. Then it is easily understood that the one cause, disturbance of normal circulation, may be the cause of many diseases occurring in different organs with entirely different symptoms.

An infection of the eye can cause impairment of sight; of the ear, impairment of hearing; of the brain, disturbances of the sensory, kinetic and mental functions; and of the joints, impairment of locomotion. But all these widely differing symptoms can be due to one and the same cause—a disturbance of the organ's blood circulation, in the form of venous congestion.

To Dr. Meyer goes credit for another discovery. Speaking before the American Geriatrics Society, he emphasized a dangerous seat of infection which has been largely overlooked—infected veins and especially jugular vein infections. He stated that teeth and tonsils spread their toxins via the small, connecting veins to the jugular veins, and from there to the rest of the body, especially the veins of the legs. As long as these venous foci are not removed, says Dr. Meyer, it is impossible to get rid of phlebitis, arthritis, and other difficulties. To correct the inflamed veins of the legs, pressure bandages are applied. To remove permanently the infection from the jugular vein, Dr. Meyer uses a method known and used since the dawn of history—the leech. In treating "jugular phlebitis" (the medical term for such inflammation) several leeches are applied over each jugular vein. Sometimes only one such treatment is required to clear up the phlebitis; in other cases two or more treatments may be necessary. As I personally have witnessed the results of this method, I present it in my Look Younger, Live Longer program. A long life is impossible as long as there are foci of infection anywhere in the body. Many authorities now recommend this treatment, among them Alton, Ochsner, Mahorner, as well as the famous Swiss ophthalmologist, Kenel. It is my hope that this simple and efficient method of removing infections of the veins will be used in the clinic of the future.

A most amazing story of leech treatment concerns the famous Australian race horse, Silent. He broke down in a race, and was retired to the country. There it was noticed that he developed a liking for a nearby leech-infested swamp and would stand in it for hours with leeches clinging to his legs. After a time the horse began to show marked improvement in health, and before long appeared to be entirely fit again. Horse sense? At any rate, from an apparently hopeless wreck, he turned again into a potential winner and was put back into training.

Of the many conditions which may be caused by venous congestion, arthritis and apoplexy, generally regarded as conditions about which little can be done, deserve to be given greater consideration. A fatalistic attitude is no longer justified, since it has been shown that in some cases arthritis can be overcome by restoring a balanced circulation in the arthritic joints, and that apoplexy can be prevented by removing the cause of congestion in the brain area.

Summarizing the treatment of infections caused by disturbances of the blood circulation, we find that the first step is to locate and remove focal infections. With these sources of infection removed, the blood stream, freed of pollution, can reestablish a balanced circulation in all organs of the body, especially when all of the vital food nutrients are used not just for a week or two, but for all the rest of your long life.

DIABETES

All diabetic diets must be supervised by the family physician. There are, however, several important nutritional discoveries from which every diabetic can benefit.

Dr. Shute and his associates in Canada, while studying heart diseases, discovered that startling results could be obtained in the treatment of diabetes by using massive doses of vitamin E. These doctors were requested to give vitamin E to an elderly man whose leg had so deteriorated with diabetic gangrene that amputation was necessary, but whose heart was too weak to withstand surgery. The vitamin E treatment was started on a Friday, at which time the patient was unable to walk. But when Dr. Shute came into the ward the following Monday, he found his patient walking around, helping the nurse serving food trays. Not only had the gangrene improved to the extent that surgery no longer was necessary, but the need for insulin was decreased and the patient's whole general condition greatly improved.

Many other physicians have now corroborated the work of

Dr. Shute and his associates. They have found that after vitamin E treatment is given, not only is the requirement of insulin often greatly reduced, but in many instances it no longer is needed, even in severe cases. Dr. Shute recommends the same massive doses of vitamin E for diabetes as he does for heart diseases.

Usually, the progress of diabetes slows down with increasing age and is controlled by a so-called "diabetic diet" which is carefully balanced as to protein, fats, and carbohydrates. Such a diet, however, is often inadequate in vitamins. For many years it has been known that a number of abnormalities can be produced in experimental laboratory animals by giving them a standard diabetic diet. Similar abnormalities can be produced in human beings on this diet, which is almost devoid of B vitamins and inadequate also in vitamins C, D, E and calcium; all of which could easily be supplied by capsules or tablets.

More serious than the diabetes itself is the possibility that diabetics sooner or later may also develop hardening of the arteries. As not all of the arteries of the body become hardened simultaneously, the blood pressure may remain normal; only the arteries of the heart or the brain or kidneys may be affected. Or sclerosis may occur in the arteries of the retina of the eye. Sometimes sclerosis develops in the arteries of the feet where it can impair circulation to the extent that gangrene develops.

If every diabetic were given some good source of B vitamins such as brewers' yeast (rich in cholin, inositol and betaine), then cholesterol would not be laid down in the arterial walls and arteriosclerosis could be prevented. Brewers' yeast, stirred into water, works well with the diabetic diet; it is almost lacking in sugar, starch and fat, yet contains 46 percent excellent protein The diabetic wishing to prevent arteriosclerosis could profit by taking at least 3 tablespoons of this yeast, daily. The B vitamins, like vitamin E, sometimes reduce the need for insulin; your doctor can be the judge of that.

Our great task in the Look Younger, Live Longer program is to *prevent* diabetes. Overeating of refined sugars and fats, for years and years, overworks and depresses the insulin-producing cells until they finally break down. I have said many times that the "human machine" is wonderfully made, but it cannot work efficiently under constant abuse. In 1900 the national consumption of white sugar was about ten pounds per person in a year. Today, what with our mountains of cheap candies and candy bars, and our oceans of soft drinks, the national average of white sugar consumed yearly is more than one hundred pounds per person.

The prevention of diabetes will be a part of the program fostered by our "human machine shops," changing the eating habits of those with diabetic tendencies and including the B vitamins and vitamin E, which Dr. Shute has proved to be so helpful.

CANCER

Much more research needs to be done on the prevention of cancer, but the growing amount of evidence points unmistakably to the fact that an adequate nutritional diet such as I have been advocating for the last thirty years is an important factor in preventing this dreaded disease.

Eat a completely adequate diet if you would guard against becoming a cancer victim. Arrange your diet so that it is relatively high in protein (lean meat, eggs, milk, fish and cheese); relatively low in carbohydrates and moderate in fats. See to it that your supply of all vitamins, especially the B vitamins, is more than adequate. Make use of such vitamin-rich nutrients as wheat germ, brewers' yeast, powdered skim milk, and yogurt, which are good sources of calcium and protein as well. Use only whole grain breads and cereals and omit all refined sugar and products containing it. Wherever possible, include foods grown on organically fertilized soil (see page 241). This last is not always easy, especially if you live in a big city. But there is proof that starved soil can only produce starved crops, and such produce can only lead to starved bodies which become easy prey to all diseases. When this fact becomes better understood, organic gardening will come into its own.

Evidence continues to accumulate that cancer follows in the path of malnutrition. Time and again, it has been pointed out that cancer is unknown among primitive peoples the world over, in Central Brazil, in Africa, in the Himalayas and other isolated spots where soils are still fertile and the milling of grains and refining of sugar are unknown. It is only when these same people adopt the diet of civilization that cancer becomes rampant. Here in our own country, the Latter-day Saints (Mormons), whose founder recommended sound dietary rules, are much freer from cancer than their fellow Americans. Experimental data indicating that poor diet is a causative factor in producing cancer is so increasingly vast that I can cite only a few examples here. Dr. J. R. Davidson of the University of Illinois has, by giving laboratory animals inadequate diets, produced cancer in 100 percent of them. Litter mates of these same animals which were kept on an adequate diet were kept free of cancer.

Experiments conducted at the University of Pennsylvania, involving one thousand animals, showed that 96 percent contracted fatal cancer when the diet was inadequate. When milk was added to the diet, fatalities were reduced to only 4 percent. When milk and all the B vitamins together were added to the diet, cancer was entirely eradicated.

At Memorial Hospital in New York, and at the University of Wisconsin, research groups showed, by tests on rats, that riboflavin (one of the B family vitamins) counteracted the effects of a cancer-causing dye which had produced liver tumors in the rats. It was also found that generous amounts of riboflavin could protect the animals against the cancerous effects of the dye.

Dietary deficiencies of proteins and B vitamins were reported as "an important predisposing cause of cancer of the mouth," at the National Cancer Conference held in Memphis, Tennessee.

More and more, reports of scientists point to the fact that research in vitamins, especially the B vitamins, plays an increasingly important role in cancer prevention work. There is also evidence that vitamins A and E are important in the prevention of cancer growth.

Dr. Albert Tannenbaum at the Medical Research Institute of the Michael Reese Hospital in Chicago has done extensive research on the relation of diet to cancer, using mice in his experiments. He discovered that overweight as well as poor diet was a serious factor. The greater incidence of cancer in the fat mice led Dr. Tannenbaum to investigate the possibility of a similarity in humans. On checking the statistical analyses of a number of insurance companies, he found that in general, the tendency to develop cancer was far greater among persons who were overweight.

From all the scientific evidence presented, we can only conclude that if the human race would keep itself "fit instead of fat" through planned nutrition, we could reduce the general incidence of cancer as well as other degenerative diseases.

And now I would like to ask a question, one that perhaps you also have wondered about. Why is it that our cancer prevention organizations, with all their drives and the huge amounts of money at their disposal, give absolutely no publicity to the important role which diet plays in the prevention of cancer?

As far back as 1942, there appeared in the *American Journal of Surgery* (New York), the following:

"Martin and Koop demonstrate from an analysis of the diets of 100 patients with precancerous stomatitis (tongue irritation), 100 with oral cancers, and 100 normal individuals, that degenerative and precancerous changes in the oral mucous membrane are among the important symptoms of deficiency diseases and also that deficiency of vitamin B is the greatest single cause of these precancerous lesions. The beneficial effects of treatment with brewers' yeast were so gratifying that the authors concluded that the abnormal changes in the oral tissues resulting from vitamin B deficiency are undoubtedly more prevalent and of more importance in the etiology of mouth cancer than any other single form of chronic irritation; possibly of greater significance than the sum total of all other factors."

With such positive statements from a reliable source, we can only hope that in our "human machine shops" of the future, when precancerous lesions are discovered, an adequate diet with optimum amounts of all the B vitamins, plus all other scientific preventatives, will be made a matter of widespread and general knowledge.

THE KIDNEYS

Like the heart, the kidneys are sturdy and can take abuse. Their performance in emergency is magnificent. If given, through adequate diet, the nutrients they require, the kidneys can be depended upon to do their share and more to function faithfully throughout a long life.

There is definite relationship between good kidney functioning and good heart functioning. The normal blood pressure of the kidneys is necessarily higher than that of other parts of the body in order to force blood plasma into the kidney tubules, in the urinary processes. An abnormally high bodily blood pressure, superimposed, over a period of years, on the already high but normal pressure in the kidneys, can readily bring about deterioration of these delicate tissues. There are also many other causes of kidney troubles, and much damage is caused by the presence of kidney stones, or gravel. In all types of experimental animals, such stones are readily produced by vitamin A deficiencies but are slowly dissolved and carried away when the vitamin again is amply supplied. Lack of vitamin A undoubtedly is one causative factor in the formation of kidney stones in human beings as well. The accumulation of minerals in the formation of kidney stones is often accelerated in vegetarian diets where too large amounts of fruits and vegetables and too little meat, eggs, milk and cereals are eaten, thus making the urine too alkaline.

Infections of the kidney can bring about destruction of the tissues, so that the walls of the kidney tubules become somewhat like a sieve, or strainer. In that event, blood proteins, which normally cannot pass into the urine, go through the damaged tubules and are lost. In normal health these proteins attract into the blood stream the waste materials from all body tissues.

When blood proteins are lost in the urine, or the diet is so deficient in protein that normal amounts of blood protein cannot be produced, liquids tend to accumulate in the body, especially in the feet, ankles and legs. When kidneys are damaged to such an extent that too much blood protein is lost and wastes cannot be collected, the result can be fatal uremic poisoning through failure to excrete uric acid.

In the prevention of kidney troubles, a high resistance to infections (discussed on page 53) must be maintained. The diet must be well planned. It must include plenty of B vitamins (brewers' yeast, for example) to keep the blood pressure normal. There must be milk and cereals to keep the urine acid, meat to supply the important blood protein, and fish-liver oil, carrots and leafy green vegetables to supply the indispensable vitamin A.

URINARY TROUBLES

Many people have the mistaken notion that it is abnormal to have to urinate during the night. On the contrary, since the bladder only holds about a quart of liquid, this is usually entirely normal; especially if quantities of liquids have been taken during the evening. Not having to urinate during the night may mean only that too small a quantity of liquids has been taken or that liquids are retained in the body tissues, or that circulation is poor.

However, the excessive urge to urinate may mean a bladder infection or irritation, incipient diabetes, or enlarged prostate. In such case, your physician should be consulted promptly so that the cause can be found and removed.

Where irritation or infection is found to exist, the dietary procedure described for treating kidney infections should be followed. Vitamins A and C must be kept extremely high; proteins should be more than adequate; and the diet should be largely of whole grain breads and cereals, meats, eggs, milk and cheese to keep the urine acid. During treatment for such irritation or infection, the use of citrus fruits and juices, and all fruits and vegetables should be largely avoided as they make the urine alkaline, a condition which allows the multiplication of bacteria. When all infections have been removed, the Live Longer diet on page 249 should be followed to prevent such troubles for the rest of your long life.

GALLSTONES

The well-known liver and gall bladder specialist, Dr. Roger Glenard of Vichy, France, has been asked thousands of times what causes some people to have constant gall bladder difficulties. His answer has become a famous saying, "Three F's contribute to gall bladder troubles: Female, Fat and Forty." It seems that women are especially prone to such troubles, often those of calm temperament, rather than the tense, nervous type.

Interestingly, psychiatrists also have pointed out that persons with "inner tensions" but with outer calmness are susceptible to gall bladder troubles. And all too often, there is also lazy elimination which can and must be corrected (see page 47).

In any case, gallstones are made up of cholesterol which is normally excreted through the bile. Under healthy conditions, the muscular wall of the gall bladder contracts sufficiently to completely empty all bile from the bladder. But when the diet lacks B vitamins, especially thiamin or B_1, normal energy is not produced and the contractions of the walls of the gall bladder become sluggish, or lacking. When the bile is not emptied, the cholesterol, being a heavy substance, settles in the stagnant bile to form gallstones. Furthermore, when the B vitamins, inositol, cholin, and betaine are lacking in the diet, the amount of cholesterol in the bile is so greatly increased that it precipitates into stones. As these stones become larger, they cannot pass through the bile duct even though the diet may have been improved and the emptying of the bladder become normal.

Those suffering with cirrhosis (fatty degeneration) of the liver are found to be especially prone to gallstones. There is an obvious connection here, in that cirrhosis of the liver also is recognized to be the result of B vitamin deficiencies, and of cholin in particular. If you have gallstones, by all means seek the advice of your physician to be rid of them.

To avoid gallstone troubles for the rest of your long life, follow the Live Longer diet on page 249. Make sure that your daily menu includes more than ample amounts of all the vital B vitamins.

DON'T BE ANEMIC

Keep your blood stream, the "river of life," flowing strongly and smoothly. Begin today to revitalize it. It needs iron and copper; the best sources of iron and copper are blackstrap molasses, wheat germ and liver. Plan to eat liver once or twice a week. Include blackstrap molasses and wheat germ in your daily meals.

Marginal anemia, a much too common complaint among people of all ages, is caused largely by an inadequate diet. Lacking iron, copper, proteins and the ever-important B vitamins, the body cannot produce enough healthy red blood cells to maintain a healthy blood stream.

Proteins are very important. As the red corpuscles contain more protein than iron, all the essential amino acids must be supplied before blood can be produced. Women in general eat less protein food than men do; therefore, low-protein anemia is more common in women than in men. This anemic condition is readily corrected when the diet contains ample amounts of the complete proteins supplied by milk, eggs, meat, wheat germ, and brewers' yeast.

All the B vitamins (thiamin, niacin, pyridoxin, para-aminobenzoic acid, folic acid, etc.) are very essential to the formation of healthy red blood cells. In particular, a lack of folic acid and of the new vitamin B_{12} appears to be the causative factor in pernicious anemia, which is one of the most serious complaints of life's later years.

Pernicious anemia (not to be confused with the commonplace marginal types) is closely connected with decreased functioning of the liver. The American scientist, George R. Minot, who discovered this connection, found that the blood vessels become saturated with immature blood cells from the bone marrow, but that the number of *red* blood cells is greatly reduced by liver disfunction, as is the total hemoglobin content.

Formerly considered incurable, pernicious anemia is now readily controlled by large doses of liver extract, providing the disease is recognized in time. Extreme cases may require blood transfusions in addition to treatment with liver extract, to reestablish more speedily a normal number of healthy red blood cells. The presence of anemia can readily be determined by a blood test which should be a routine part of your regular medical examination.

To help you plan an adequate diet, rich in all the nutrients needed to prevent or overcome anemia, remember that liver, wheat germ, and blackstrap molasses are natural sources of proteins, iron, copper, and B vitamins which the blood needs. Liver and wheat germ are rich sources of the B vitamins, folic acid and

B₁₂, and should be cooked no longer than five or ten minutes to retain the full value of these essential nutrients. Fortunately for those with pernicious anemia, folic acid and vitamin B₁₂ are now available in concentrated form and only a few milligrams a day have saved many a sufferer from this heretofore mysterious disease.

VARICOSE VEINS

Although the beating, or pumping action, of the heart forces the blood throughout the body, its effect diminishes as the blood passes into the thousands of miles of capillaries. The return of the blood to the heart is brought about by contractions of muscles; the back flow of the blood toward the arteries is prevented by valves in the veins. If, however, the muscles fail to contract normally, the blood cannot be pushed on in its return to the heart. Then blood stays in the veins; it clots and remains there. Other blood may be pushed into the clogged veins and if not forced out will likewise remain to form clots. Such clogged veins, filled with stagnant blood, are spoken of as varicose veins. In time, new blood vessels are formed around the plugged veins, but the varicosities themselves remain to become unsightly, perhaps painful, and in extreme cases ulcerous.

There are two methods for removing unsightly varicosities. One is by surgery, which eliminates the difficulty permanently and is a comparatively simple operation, but requires hospitalization. The other is the injection method which has become very popular in Europe and in America. Discuss these methods with your doctor if you are troubled with varicosities; do not spend the second half of life trying to hide them. And do remember that unless the diet is improved and the muscular tone strengthened, more enlarged veins are apt to appear.

The problem of *preventing* varicose veins becomes one of maintaining healthy muscle tone with muscles so strong and elastic that, as they contract, they will completely squeeze the blood from the veins passing through them. Since muscles are made of protein, they can maintain their strength only when generous amounts of adequate protein are eaten. Protein in the diet should be increased when any varicose veins appear. Such high protein foods as powdered skim milk, wheat germ, and brewers' yeast should be used liberally in addition to a quart of liquid milk daily, one or two eggs, a serving each of cheese and meat.

It has been found that varicose veins develop ulcers when protein is inadequate and will heal only when generous amounts of protein are obtained. The healing of such ulcers also is hastened by taking liberal amounts of vitamin C. A well-balanced diet, such as our Look Younger, Live Longer diet on page 249, is the best possible preventative for varicose veins.

MENTAL DISTURBANCES

I am never happier than when I find that the science of nutrition is becoming more and more helpful in preventing mental deterioration and disease. Mental disease does not "just happen"; it is the end product of a long series of causative factors. Happily, some of these causes are simply nutritional; *these can be eradicated*.

It has long been known that a severe lack of the B vitamin, niacin, can result in dementia, or insanity. Furthermore, when human volunteers have been kept on diets lacking almost any one of the B vitamins, it led to the development of mental confusion, depression and anxiety states.

When Dr. Sydenstricker, in his studies, kept human volunteers on a diet adequate in all respects except for the B vitamin, biotin, the resultant mental depression became so severe that his subjects developed suicidal tendencies and the experiments had to be stopped. Such findings indicate that lack of the B vitamins may well be a causative factor in inducing insanity, or at least be a forerunner of mental collapse.

Groups of scientists, particularly in Sweden, have studied the brains of persons who died insane and have compared them with the brains of normal individuals who met accidental death. They found that four substances essential to the healthy nucleus of brain cells were lacking in the insane; adenine, thymine, cytosine and quanine. These four nutrients are found in multicellular meats such as liver, calf or lamb brains, sweetbreads, kidneys, and in brewers' yeast. Such excellent meats should be eaten frequently, and brewers' yeast should be added to the daily diet.

Statistics show that one out of every twenty persons spends some time of his life in an institution for mental diseases. *Let us change these shocking statistics.* How? By proclaiming a dietary revolution. Hand in hand with the ever-developing science of psychiatry, the science of nutrition can work toward the prevention of mental illness. It can give mankind the freedom he longs for, freedom from the greatest of all his fears—the fear of losing his mind.

NERVOUSNESS

Eat and stop fidgeting. Nervousness is often a result of unwise diet. That high-strung, jittery feeling, that jingle-jangle of nerves, is largely your body's protest against an undersupply of calcium and the vital B vitamins.

Calcium, of which fortified milk is the best source, is essential for serenity. If you want to do away with the jitters, learn to drink a quart of milk daily, preferably fortified with half a cup of powdered skim milk well beaten into it and with vitamin D added to ensure the efficient absorption of the calcium. If you are especially high-strung, it would also be wise to take calcium tablets combined with vitamin D before meals and at bedtime.

Scientific experiments with human volunteers have shown that diets lacking any one or several of the B vitamins can quickly produce nervous tension. A serious lack of vitamin B_6 (pyridoxin) has even resulted in muscular tremors and uncontrollable shaking of the hands or head. The importance of this vitamin cannot be overemphasized in view of the fact that such serious diseases as palsy (paralysis agitans), St. Vitus dance and epilepsy have shown marked improvement with the dietary addition of adequate B_6.

A planned, adequate diet is essential to calmness and a vibrant sense of well-being. On page 249 I have outlined a diet containing all the nutrients necessary to sound nerves in a sound body.

In older people, fidgets and a sense of fatigue often result from so simple a thing as failure to eat *between* meals, when the blood sugar drops below normal. Without adequate natural blood sugar, energy is not produced, food fats are not completely burned, and a feeling of nervousness results. This can be quickly overcome by a small mid-meal of fruit or fruit juices; a glass of milk; some cheese and crackers, or any snack containing small amounts of starch and natural sugars.

In the light of scientific evidence, and personal observation, it is my belief that adherence to a well-planned nutritional diet, plus the ability to relax all parts of the body, would eliminate an infinite variety of "nerves" for which the pace of our modern world conveniently takes the blame. Remember that it is impossible to be tense and nervous when the body is relaxed.

To Look Younger and Live Longer, you must be free from "nerves." Learn as much as you can about their cause, about the general laws of mind and body and about your own mental quirks. If necessary, go to a trained psychotherapist and let him help you uncover those trouble-making parts of your personality which you cannot find and correct yourself.

FORGETFULNESS

Stella Nash, who likes the form of headgear known as a beanie, went into the kitchen, beanie in hand, to get a glass of milk from the refrigerator. She drank the milk, carried the emptied milk bottle to the hall closet. "Where on earth is my beanie?" she asked, several hours later, turning the hall closet upside down. The beanie was in the refrigerator.

- Stella is "getting on," you say? Beginning to be absent-minded? Stella is sixteen. It was her mother who told me the story. Mrs. Nash, a delightful woman in her mid-forties, had gone to the hall closet for a suit that needed cleaning. Seeing the milk bottle her daughter had absent-mindedly left there, she picked it up—and absent-mindedly handed it, instead of the suit, to the waiting dry-cleaner's man!

Absent-mindedness is a sign of something, psychologists tell us, but it is not necessarily a sign of old age. It can be a sign of dietary deficiency.

One of the Philadelphia hospitals conducted tests for memory, clarity, speed of thinking, and general intelligence among a group of elderly patients living on a standard hospital diet. The tests were made before and after a number of the B vitamins were separately given them, and repeated again when the entire B family was amply supplied by natural foods. There was no change in native intelligence, but the patients showed improvement in memory and ability to think clearly after the separate B vitamins were given. Marked improvement followed, however, when *all* of the B vitamins were amply supplied. Anyone who has difficulty in remembering or who finds his thinking growing foggy and confused, will usually notice that same marked improvement in himself when he adds such food nutrients as brewers' yeast and wheat germ to his diet.

Recent experimental work has shown that one of the amino acids, known as glutamic acid, is a principal component of an enzyme in the brain. When glutamic acid is amply supplied in the diet, the intelligence has been found to be actually increased, the ability to learn is accelerated, thinking is clearer, and memory becomes more keen and accurate. While glutamic acid is found in all complete proteins, it is interesting to note that the protein of milk (lactalbumin) is more than 50 percent glutamic acid. Fresh and powdered milk and cheeses of all kinds are therefore the best sources of this invaluable nutrient.

If you are forgetful, absent-minded, or slow on the uptake, do not say, "It's my age," and let it go at that. Follow the Live Longer diet outlined on page 249; it is rich in proteins and B vitamins. It will send you frequently to the refrigerator to get a glass of fortified milk, and help you remember where you put your hat.

ALLERGIES, HAY FEVER AND ASTHMA

Allergies usually appear when health is below par and as frequently disappear when a sound nutritional program is followed long enough to result in a general improvement in health. In correcting allergies, the emphasis should not be on one or two nutrients, but on a diet adequate in all respects.

Vitamin C appears to detoxify foreign materials which get into the blood, hence it is of particular importance in preventing or treating allergies. The person who has a history of allergies should take at least 100 milligrams of vitamin C at each meal, in tablet form, if it is not readily available in foods. During a severe allergic attack, relief is often gained by taking 100 milligrams of vitamin C every one or two hours.

In cases where the mucous membranes are affected, as in hay fever or other allergies which cause congestion of the sinuses and nasal passages, large amounts of vitamin A are indicated. Vitamin A is particularly important in building the health of the mucous membranes, and as much as 50,000 units should be taken after each meal until the allergy disappears. Where hay fever habitually appears at a certain time each year, the taking of 150,000 units of vitamin A daily for two months prior to the expected attack will usually prevent it, provided that the diet is adequate in all other respects as well.

In asthma, the difficulty in breathing is brought on by spasms of the diaphragm. Relaxation is effected and the spasms relieved or prevented when calcium is adequately supplied. During a severe asthmatic attack, two or three calcium tablets should be taken every hour, and at all other times calcium should be kept adequate by using milk and milk products generously. It must be remembered that vitamin D is necessary before calcium can be absorbed or utilized; therefore be sure that the calcium tablets you take also contain vitamin D.

A rather new treatment for asthma which appears to hold promise is that of using large amounts of vitamin E. It is known that vitamin E decreases the need for oxygen in the body. Asthma attacks frequently follow violent exertion, when the need for oxygen is increased, or when the oxygen supply is decreased as in high altitudes and in rainy or foggy weather. The amount of vitamin E given is the same as that used in treating heart disease, discussed on page 37.

To overcome allergies, be sure to follow the Live Longer diet (see page 249), rich in all nutrients to keep your vitality high for the rest of your long life. In no other circumstance have such inadequate diets been recommended as those generally used in treating food allergies. For example, if the patient is allergic to milk he is told to avoid it and immediately becomes deficient in proteins, calcium, and vitamin B_2. In such case, canned milk, powdered milk or yogurt can often be tolerated well and these foods should certainly be tried. For every food foregone, the nutrients supplied by that food must be furnished by a substitute food if health is to be maintained.

PSYCHOSOMATIC DIFFICULTIES

"Psycho" refers to the mind and "somo" to the body; "psychosomatic" therefore refers to the relationship and reaction of mind and body, one to the other. In recent years, much has been written about psychosomatic difficulties. We have all become increasingly aware that worries, emotional upsets and anxieties can have such a tremendous effect upon general health that they can be causative factors in producing severe illnesses.

Such abnormalities as asthma, hay fever and other allergies, migraine headaches, digestive disturbances, diarrhea, and high blood pressure may have several causes. All, however, *can* be induced by psychosomatic disturbances.

The point which I feel has been *almost wholly overlooked* in the annals of psychosomatic medicine is the role of *B vitamin deficiencies* in producing the original emotional problems at the root of such disturbances. It is just now being recognized that anxiety states develop when the diet contains too little of the several B vitamins, particularly B_1 (thiamin), niacin, and biotin. These anxiety states are characterized by excessive worrying and brooding, mental depression, emotional instability and nervous tensions.

The person suffering psychosomatic illness frequently has allowed himself to develop multiple deficiencies of the B vitamins to such extent that he is readily upset emotionally. If an allergy also has developed, and a restricted diet supplying even less of the B vitamins is followed, the whole psychosomatic condition becomes worse. A vicious circle then has been set up, for which the obvious correction is to plan a complete diet adequate in all respects and extremely high in all the B vitamins. Such a diet would include, daily, several heaping tablespoonfuls of brewers' yeast; half a cup of wheat germ; one tablespoon or more of blackstrap molasses; and from a pint to a quart of yogurt.

BRITTLE BONES

Bones need not become brittle and fragile with age. Such brittle bones are only the accumulative result of eating foods so deficient in nutrients that bone strength could not be maintained. It has been found in experiments with laboratory animals that where the diet has been entirely adequate the bones become harder and *stronger* with age.

To maintain healthy bones for a lifetime, you must eat foods adequate in all nutrients. Sufficient calcium and phosphorus are essential. These minerals are not readily absorbed into the blood stream nor deposited in the bones *unless* vitamin D is supplied with them. And as vitamin D does not occur in many foods, it must be obtained from some form of fish-liver oil.

The cartilage-like base of the bones, made up of protein, breaks down whenever there is a lack, or undersupply, of protein nutrients or any of the essential amino acids. And these protein cells are cemented together by an elastic substance, collagen, which depends upon vitamin C for its tenacity and elasticity.

If the daily diet is planned to supply adequately all of these vital nutrients (calcium, phosphorus, proteins, vitamins D and C) there need be no fear of broken bones at any age, nor question of delayed healing should broken bones occur. Thousands of people have wasted their later years in wheelchairs because of incompletely healed fractures, blaming it on "old age" and never knowing that their diet was at fault.

ARTHRITIS

There are two forms of arthritis: infectious and chronic. The infectious form of arthritis, which produces serious disability, is not caused by any one factor but by many. And the seat of the infection, whether teeth, tonsils, jugular vein (see Dr. Meyer's treatment for infections on page 59), or other source must be cleared up before health can be regained. Then sound nutrition will play a vital part in full recovery.

Another new note of hope for those suffering arthritis has

been sounded by Dr. Walter Bauer of the Harvard Medical School, and by Dr. Philip S. Hench of the Mayo foundation. Injections of a hormone from the adrenal gland were found to bring dramatic relief to a number of their patients. But the thousands of arthritic sufferers are warned not to pin their entire hopes on this, as it is still in the experimental field and much more research work must be done.

There is also good news for arthritics in the Mayo Clinic report on a new hormone called Cortisone or Compound E, which has shown spectacular results in the treatment of rheumatoid arthritis. More recently, another hormone made from the pituitary glands of hogs has been used with almost miraculous benefit. These magic hormones can be extracted from certain plants in quantities large enough to put them within reach of all who need such treatment.

In experimental laboratories, arthritis has been produced in animals by depriving them of vitamin C over a period of weeks and then injecting bacteria into them. The bacteria were carried throughout the body and spilled into the small joints first; there the body tried desperately to stop the infection by depositing calcium all around it. Pain and swelling developed, and arthritic stiffness followed. On the other hand, where animals had been on a balanced diet with optimum amounts of vitamin C, the injected bacteria did not enter the blood stream but caused an abscess to form at the point of injection. When the abscess broke, the dangerous bacteria were promptly expelled and of course there was no arthritis. The lesson to be learned from this is: Do not tolerate any infection anywhere in the body. Consult your doctor immediately.

Our Look Younger, Live Longer diet is the best possible insurance against arthritic difficulties. Do use maximum amounts of vitamin C daily, say one 100-milligram tablet after each meal. Get plenty of protective proteins, especially lean meats, cheese, and a quart of fortified yogurt to help produce antibodies in the blood stream. Use only whole grain breads and cereals, and eat moderate amounts of fruits and vegetables. Calcium is very important, and should never be restricted as it was in old-fashioned incomplete diets.

MENOPAUSE

The really healthy woman finds the menopause as free of difficulty as was the experience of puberty. She is aware only that the ovaries become less active and cease to bring about the conditions necessary to conception. And few, indeed, are the women over forty who would wish to continue bearing children.

Menopause difficulties often indicate that the diet has been inadequate, and usually can be stopped or prevented with adherence to a normal, adequate diet. Hot flashes, night sweats, extreme tensions, nervousness, and insomnia tend to disappear when more than the minimum daily amounts of calcium and the B vitamins are added. Physicians often recommend that one or two calcium tablets, or mixed mineral tablets supplying calcium deficiencies, be taken before meals and at bedtime. Vitamin D, usually deficient in diets, should also be included. It is necessary in the absorption and efficient utilization of calcium.

Irregular flowing has been found to correct itself when all the B vitamins are supplied through daily use of brewers' yeast, wheat germ and blackstrap molasses. Excessive flowing and many other symptoms will in many cases disappear when 30 to 60 milligrams of vitamin E are taken after each meal. For the woman who suffers excessive flowing, I would also advise a thorough medical examination to rule out the possibility of fibroid growths which often develop in the uterus.

Recent reports indicate a growing use of vitamin E in treating menopausal difficulties, especially where hormone treatment cannot be given for one reason or another. Just before the war, two British physicians reported that the use of vitamin E had successfully quieted menopausal flushes and sweats. Recollection of this report proved immensely valuable to two doctors interned with other war prisoners in a Japanese camp in the Philippines. They lacked hormone supplies, but did have a quantity of vitamin E in the form of wheat germ oil. For the many women prisoners suffering menopausal troubles, the vitamin E treatment proved extremely beneficial. After the war, another doctor investigated the benefits of vitamin E in treating a large group of women in the menopause. His report stated that the entire group "showed a dramatic response; there was great relief from the drenching perspiration, frequency and intensity of hot flashes, and marked change in mood and outlook."

Judging from these reports, while treatment of the menopausal syndrome is a medical problem, the prevention of it very obviously lies in the field of nutrition. You can be sure that your diet supplies adequate amounts of vitamin E by using wheat germ; by adding wheat germ oil to your salad dressings; and by using only whole wheat bread and cereals, whole rye, brown rice, and whole buckwheat. The unsaturated fatty acids supplied by wheat germ oil, important to vitamin E, are also richly found in vegetable oils but are not present in prepared shortening, butter and margarine. (See page 276 for salad dressing and other vitamin E recipes.)

An all too frequent accompaniment of the menopause is the

anemic condition brought about by an inadequate diet during the years of natural loss of iron and copper through menstruation. Blackstrap molasses, wheat germ and liver are the richest sources of iron and copper and should be added liberally to the diet. With daily use of the first two, and liver once or twice a week, the woman suffering menopausal anemia should experience rapid recovery.

Sufficient proteins are also important to the body in overcoming menopausal anemia and building up the body for a long and healthy life. Ample amounts of the complete proteins supplied by milk, eggs, meat, wheat germ, and brewers' yeast must be made a part of your planned nutrition program. On page 249 you will find the Live Longer Diet Plan containing all these essential nutrients.

Many of the "problems" of the menopause actually are only coincidental; many are brought about by fear. Throughout the ages, unhealthy and neurotic women have made the most of any symptoms which appear at menopause in order to gain self-importance and sympathetic attention. Their tales of woe have made many otherwise healthy women fearful of what may be expected at that period.

For the healthy woman, sexual desire does not end with the end of the reproductive functions. It can continue indefinitely, and with adjustment to the menopause she can embark upon a new life that is satisfactory and harmonious. Moreover, freed from the fear of unwanted pregnancy and other problems of menstruation, the well-adjusted and healthy woman is pleased to have her energies freed for the many other interests and activities of life.

All too often, both men and women mistakenly believe that a woman's capacity for sexual feeling disappears after the meno pause. They quite fail to realize that her sexual feelings come from many sources which are in no way affected by decreased ovarian activity. Contrary to their mistaken beliefs, a woman's sexual enjoyment may be greatly increased after menopause.

Loving and being loved is the fundamental human experience, essential to the formation of character and a positive attitude toward life. Sex is both spiritual and physical; from a mutual exchange of affection emerges tenderness and affection which bring health and harmony and enhance the total personality. Longevity statistics indicate conclusively that older people who are happily married have the best chance of achieving a healthy long life.

If false sex education has given you latent hangovers of guilt, or if the constrictive influence of possessive parents has created a problem, have no hesitation in discussing such problems fully and openly with your doctor or psychiatrist, and be guided accordingly. Know that thousands upon thousands of other humans have had such troubles and have overcome them. Know also that sex is a natural and normal function, that it can be one of life's greatest blessings for both men and women.

In any case, it is important to give your body a health-building, adequate diet especially rich in calcium, the vitamins B, D and E. Should any unpleasant menopausal symptoms linger, consult an endocrinologist. Medical science has now perfected glandular therapy to the point where it can deal swiftly with abnormal menopausal problems. With the endocrinologist's aid and your health-building diet, you soon will discover that your *change* in life becomes your *chance* in life.

It is my conviction that the whole bugaboo of menopausal troubles could be dispelled for all time if our overcivilized diets gave way to planned nutritional diets. The forethought of an adequate diet, begun with our first spoonful of food, would obviate the need for afterthought in our later years.

YOU CAN FEED YOUR GLANDS

Some years ago, on the terrace of the San Francisco Yacht Club, I lunched with Gertrude Atherton, author of the memorable novel about rejuvenation, *Black Oxen*. Mrs. Atherton talked frankly and forthrightly about the subject, and told me that she herself had taken rejuvenation treatments from Dr. Harry Benjamin, a pupil of the famous Dr. Steinach in Vienna. She also said that since writing *Black Oxen*, she had been deluged with mail from all over the world, from prematurely aging men and women asking for help. In talking about my work as a nutritionist, and my conviction that planned diet can do much to prevent aging and premature senility, she urged me to "let the whole world know of it—spread that knowledge far and wide." And right there, she planted the seed for this book.

The more I study, and practice, and observe, the more convinced I become that planned nutrition can prevent premature aging. Looking younger and living longer depend in great measure on the harmonious functioning of all your glands, and you can feed your glands. A great amount of research has been done, and more is needed, but today there is definite proof that with the food we eat from day to day, we can do a lot for our glands. The natural path to a longer, healthier and happier life is via scientific nutrition.

Dr. Louis Berman, famous endocrinologist, wrote that he looked forward to the day when mankind would change its attitude toward food—would regard it not as foreign matter to be ingested by the stomach, but as something about to become an integral part of oneself, which it surely is. The food you eat affects your character and personality through the functioning of your glands. The continuous interaction of all the glands regulates the light in your eyes, the beauty of your smile, spiritual radiance, clarity of mind, precision of thought, atmosphere of presence, bodily courage, facial lines, emotions and voice, general behavior and manner.

The glands themselves are made of protein and their youthifying secretions, the hormones, also are protein. The hormones go directly into the blood stream and are the important "directors" of all the chemical processes of the entire body. A lack of protein can readily weaken all glandular functions and thus cause premature aging. Adequate minerals and vitamins also are necessary to maintain a healthy balance in the functioning of your glands. It is not by accident that the gay, the cheerful, the wise and hopeful ones live longer and happier lives than the depressed, the envious, the gossips, the worriers and the fanatics; it is the natural result of balanced, harmonious glandular functions stemming from balanced, adequate nutrition.

Endocrinology is an absorbing study, and many fascinating books have been written by many scientists, but the thing which impresses me most is the fact that the glands of internal secretion are all dependent upon one another to create a symphony of hormones which bring life and health to every cell in the body. The famous Voronoff transplant was made, not with just one gland, but with a combination of the pituitary, the thyroid and the sex glands. These are the ones which have received the most intensive study during the last fifty years, and I shall write of them in greater detail, and of the foods, vitamins and minerals needed to keep our own glands healthy and smoothly functioning.

THE PITUITARY GLAND

Weighing only six-tenths of a gram, it is located just back of the nose and beneath the brain, but small as it is, the pituitary has been termed the "director" of the entire "glandular symphony." This tiny gland manufactures ten or more hormones which are tremendously important in their effect upon every other gland in the body. One of its hormones directs the growth of bones and tissues; through its sex hormone it directs sex stimulation and the activities of the ovaries. It controls the thyroid gland and the insulin-producing gland (the pancreas). It even controls formation of fat, and where the fat shall be deposited in the body.

One of the diseases of the pituitary gland which endocrinologists encounter frequently is an excess of fat deposited around the chest and abdomen in a girdle-like fashion. Men take on female characteristics, and women become somewhat masculine; the sex glands become smaller and the sex life gradually diminishes. Often, such fat people are only too ready to blame their glands and do nothing about it. The truth of the matter is that for years they have been overeating on fats and carbohydrates, overworking and weakening the glands (especially the pituitary) which strive to maintain a balance against impossible odds. Only the right diet—and I'll emphasize that—can prevent or overcome this type of bulky fat.

Dr. Newburg of the University of Michigan has shown that even extremely fat people with serious glandular problems (like the fat lady in the circus) can reduce to normal weight, and their glandular functions be returned to normal, by means of a carefully selected diet and without glandular therapy. The fat person who sighs, "It's my glands," and reaches for another helping of fattening food, no longer has a scientific leg to stand upon. While glandular therapy can be invaluable, "glandular shots" alone can never completely correct obesity; a scientifically selected diet is of prime importance.

When the pituitary gland does not function properly, it adversely affects the ovaries and brings about premature menopause. It is interesting to note that whereas underfunction of the pituitary produces an earlier menopause, the underfunctioning of the thyroid causes a later-than-normal menopause.

Here are the foods necessary to the all-important pituitary gland. First class proteins: meat, eggs, cheese and fortified milk. Meat especially seems to have a stimulating effect. Foods high in manganese: wheat germ, liver, potatoes and nuts. Wheat germ also is rich in vitamin E, which the pituitary uses in greater amounts than any other gland of the body. All vitamins; but especially those of the B family, of which the richest sources are yogurt, wheat germ, brewers' yeast. (Also see menus on page 249.)

THE THYROID GLAND

This gland lies in the foreground of the throat, astride the windpipe, and has been called the "watchman" between the physical and mental body. The thyroid secretes a liquid which is constantly poured into the blood stream and carried to all parts of the body. Removal or disability of the thyroid can turn a youthful person into an old one. Dr. G. W. Crile, who has done much research with the thyroid, discovered that it secretes hormones which give the body much of its verve and virility.

A weak or lazy thyroid can make the sex glands lazy, and an overactive thyroid overstimulates the sex glands. The great Don

Juans you read about are the overactive thyroid type, and the indifferent lovers usually have a lazy thyroid.

One of the important functions of the thyroid is the burning of fat, and an underactive thyroid can cause much unnecessary fat to be deposited all over the body (not just in girdle fashion, as with the pituitary type). The hormone secreted which regulates metabolism and the burning of fat is called thyroxin, and is largely made up of iodine. And the lack of iodine in our over-refined foods is responsible for much thyroid trouble, from simple goiter to myxedema.

Mental sluggishness, difficulty in remembering, and the constant desire to sleep are typical problems of thyroid starvation. The thyroid has so many important functions in keeping us slim, trim and alert, in keeping the hair, nails and complexion healthy, that it could also be termed the "beauty master" of the body. Not only can wrong diet disturb the balance of this sensitive gland, but the resultant depression, fear and worry and constant strain can further weaken it. Fortunately, a great deal is now known about this gland and many difficulties once thought to be incurable now can be permanently corrected.

Adequate iodine is of foremost importance for normal, healthy functioning of the thyroid. Without it, we grow old before our time, are always tired, and wonder whatever became of our usual pep. Without essential iodine, we may find ourselves becoming soft and flabby of flesh; mentally lazy and unable to take much interest in anything; lapsing into the blues; and never feeling warm enough, especially in the hands and feet.

Dr. Russell Wilder of the Mayo Foundation has found that when human volunteers do not get sufficient vitamin B_1, the thyroid gland becomes inactive, the basal metabolism drops far below normal; and that the condition was not corrected by giving thyroid extract. It was corrected by giving vitamin B₁ without any thyroid. Probably thousands of people who now take thyroid extract would be far more helped by following a diet rich in all the B vitamins.

Here, then, are the essential foods for a well-balanced, smoothly functioning thyroid. First class proteins: meat, eggs, cheese and fortified milk. Abundant iodine: shrimps, oysters, salmon, radishes, tomatoes, watercress, sea greens and cod liver oil and iodized vegetable salt. All the B vitamins, which are richly contained in brewers' yeast, yogurt, wheat germ and blackstrap molasses. And for the rest of your long life, season all foods with iodized salt, preferably iodized vegetable salt.

THE PARATHYROID GLANDS

These are tiny oval glands located at each side of the thyroid, so small that the average number (4) have a total weight of about half a gram. Our chief interest in the parathyroids is the fact that they regulate the bodily supply of calcium, distributing it throughout the body and, when necessary, extracting it from one place to supply another—"robbing Peter to pay Paul." If the calcium level in the blood stream decreases, it may cause strange allergies, painful cramps, and spasms. Serious deficiencies or an imbalance of calcium and phosphorus are associated with neurotic conditions; adequate calcium is essential to maintaining calm nerves, as well as to the building of strong healthy bones and teeth.

To keep the mighty little parathyroids functioning properly, get plenty of calcium-rich foods such as fortified milk and cheese. Take tablets of calcium with vitamin D, which is essential to the complete utilization of the calcium. Consult the menus on page 356 for other high calcium foods, and remember that sunshine is a potent source of essential vitamin D.

THE ADRENALS

There are two of these glands, weighing only half an ounce, and located one atop each kidney like little caps. The adrenals produce the hormone, adrenalin, which is poured into the blood stream in time of danger or strong emotional upheaval, to brace us for action or to sustain shock. A deficiency of adrenalin causes slowed-down reactions. The adrenal glands also have power to destroy many poisons and free the body from dangerous toxins, and have been termed "the glands of survival." While much remains to be learned about these glands, it has been found that nicotine, lead, and other chemicals can cause them great damage, and that an unbalanced diet is definitely injurious. It is also suspected that malfunctioning of these glands plays a part in graying of the hair.

In addition to first class proteins, the diet for healthy adrenal glands must contain sufficient salt, vitamins A, C, and the B family. Vitamin C helps in the elimination of poisons; vitamin A prevents congestions; and the B vitamins are vital to the production of adrenalin. On page 349 I have listed a variety of foods supplying these essential nutrients.

THE PANCREAS

As is well known, this gland manufactures the hormone we call insulin, whose chief purpose is to help the body utilize and store sugar, or glycogen. When the pancreas becomes damaged and no longer secretes insulin, sugar is lost in the urine, and we have diabetes. This vital gland, which is several inches long, lies across the middle of the abdominal cavity. In addition to the production of insulin, it pours enzymes into the upper intestine for the digestion of proteins, fats, sugars, and starches.

While the exact cause, or causes, of diabetes is not entirely known, we have proof that the overeating of sugars and fats overworks the pancreas, and after years of such abuse it finally breaks down and stops producing insulin. (See discussion of diabetes on page 61.) Optimum amounts of all the B vitamins can help an overworked or abused pancreas to produce more insulin. In addition to B vitamin foods, such rich sources as yogurt, wheat germ, and brewers' yeast should be added to the diet. A half cup of wheat germ daily, or a heaping tablespoonful of brewers' yeast, both of which are practically starch-free, can be very beneficial to the diabetic.

THE SEX GLANDS

"Yet all were lacking if sex were lacking," said Walt Whitman, and one cannot deny the importance of a well-regulated and controlled sex life. Most people, however, do not realize that the sex glands also have other functions and purposes. According to the famous Dr. Steinach, both the male and female sex glands have two distinctly different functions; they produce internal as well as external secretions. The external secretion, as we all know, produces human offspring, whereas the internal secretion revitalizes your own body. It is continuation of this inner revitalization which becomes so important to us in the second half of life, since it perpetuates our own vitality and wellbeing. Dr. Steinach created a furor in Vienna (and all over the world) by applying this principle to aging men. The famous Steinach operation—a relatively simple procedure for men—consists in tying up the vas deferens duct to prevent ejaculation of secretions, and thus diverting them to increasing the bodily vigor. This simple operation, which takes about twenty minutes, has benefited many, and Dr. Adolph Lorenz has testified openly to its beneficial effects. However, as this is a very personal problem, if you have further interest in it I suggest consulting your own physician.

Our chief interest here is in how to keep the sex glands healthy via the most reliable and most permanent way—sound nutrition. A basically well-balanced diet is the first step toward improvement of the sex glands, as it is with all glands. When nutritional deficiencies have been overcome, improved health and vigor will be reflected in greater virility and normal libido. Remember that first class proteins as well as vitamins A, C, E, and all the B vitamins (especially pantothenic acid, para-aminobenzoic acid, and folic acid) are imperative for glandular health. The virility and longevity of the Bulgarians is probably due in great measure to the daily eating of yogurt, because the yogurt bacillus has the fortunate ability to synthesize the B vitamins in the intestine. Vitamin A is needed for the health of the ovaries and the prostate, and controls the rhythm of the sexual cycle. Vitamin E is needed for the formation of sperm.

A general degeneration of the sex glands follows upon an undersupply of almost any of the B vitamins, but is most rapid and severe when pantothenic acid is deficient. Progressive sexual inactivity develops when too little iron or vitamin C is supplied. Vitamin E, however, seems to have a very marked effect on the sex glands and is essential for the health of both ovaries and testicles. A loss of sex interest occurs in severe deficiencies of this vitamin, and the complete lack of vitamin E can result in irreparable sterility in the male.

When the ovaries do not function properly, a type of fat is deposited on the breasts and upper thighs, usually at middle age. While glandular therapy can be of great help in such cases, a sound reducing diet (see page 301) is necessary to be rid of such fat permanently.

In men, fear and worry may be the worst troublemakers in preventing normal sexual functioning, especially in later years. And such fears and worries may be brought on by a lack of B vitamins as much as by a man's own erroneous beliefs concerning sex. How often, and how wrongly, the man views an active sex life as the symbol of youth. Medical records show that libido, the ability to have intercourse, and the production of living semen sometimes are sustained up to a very great age, and that frustration will create all the unpleasant neurotic symptoms of any forced abstinence. Actually, the need for sexual outlet is an individual matter depending entirely upon the make-up of each individual person. No standard patterns can be set up for what might be called normal or average sex activity for all.

Sexual emotion depends upon the amount of internal secretions delivered to the blood by the gonads. These in turn must depend upon the amount of nutrients available to maintain the health of the ovaries and testicles. People who have lived on inadequate or starvation diets (as did those in concentration camps) invariably report that sex interest quickly and completely disappeared.

Animals maintained on diets low in protein, or inadequate in any of the essential amino acids, show so little sex interest that mating soon ceases. On a high protein diet, restoration of sexual potency and the resumption of mating are quickly resumed. The importance of a diet adequate in all nutrients in maintaining sexual potency cannot be overemphasized. A lack of the amino acid, arginine, causes sterility in male animals. In experiments with young men it was shown that inadequate arginine, over a period of only one week, resulted in a marked decrease in sperm production.

The studies of Reynolds and Macomber showed that calcium deficiency had the same effect as that of protein starvation. Too little vitamin A can cause a marked reduction in fertility, disturbed sexual behavior, and, in severe cases, complete loss of libido.

Should any of your endocrine glands not function properly, the first step is to follow a balanced diet rich in all the important nutrients, the Live Longer diet as outlined on page 249. As the entire bodily nutrition improves, glandular difficulties should disappear. If trouble continues, probably as the result of long neglect, by all means consult the best endocrinologist in your locality and get to the root of the trouble. With present-day knowledge of the glands, and the aid of highly scientific glandular preparations, your endocrinologist is well equipped to bring back to health weakened or malfunctioning glands.

I believe that, with our ever-increasing understanding of the glands and their vital secretions, we are about to enter the "Hormone Age," and I predict that the day is not distant when diets rich in hormone-producing vitamins, to protect our life-giving and life-sustaining glands against depletion and disease, will be the general rule rather than the exception.

VI. OVERWEIGHT? JOIN EATERS ANONYMOUS

NEXT TO ALCOHOLICS, overeaters are the greatest alibi artists on earth. They kid themselves unmercifully; unless they face their weakness, they are capable, quite literally, of kidding themselves to death. The alcoholic takes his poison in the form of excessive foodless carbohydrates contained in alcohol. The overeater takes his poison in the form of excessive carbohydrates contained in foodless starches and sugars.

We hear a great deal nowadays about alcoholism—that it is a malady, a symptom of personal maladjustment to life. We hear that a good way to cure it is for alcoholics to admit that they cannot drink moderately, decide to stop drinking entirely, and get together with other reformed alcoholics for moral support.

We do not hear so much about overeating. Overeaters are not public nuisances; they do not estrange their families; they do not argue with cops and land in jail. Of course, they look and feel like the deuce—lots older than they actually are. Three chins and fifty to one hundred pounds of excess fat never made anybody dashing, youthful, or glamorous. Also, they are undoubtedly shortening their lives. Insurance companies agree that, for *every inch* you let your waistline exceed your chest line, you shorten your life by *one year*.

In our Look Younger, Live Longer program, we deplore excessive drinking and are heartily in sympathy with the widespread efforts being made by doctors, psychiatrists, and thoughtful people everywhere to understand alcoholism and help alcoholics understand and help themselves.

We see America plagued by another malady—overeating. We see millions of people eating themselves into bodily misery and early graves, cheating themselves and their families of the best and happiest and most productive years of their lives. Therefore, with a salute to Alcoholics Anonymous, a nationwide movement which we admire tremendously, we have launched a nationwide movement of our own—Eaters Anonymous. Eaters Anonymous invites every American who cannot eat moderately to admit it, decide to stop overeating, and get together with other reformed overeaters for moral support.

Why do people tend to overeat, as they grow older?

From habit, as often as not. Eating is the first habit we form in life. Hunger is our first drive, its satisfaction our earliest pleasure. Later, other drives and other pleasures may put eating in the background. But as people grow older they are under less pressure from other drives; they expect (mistakenly) less satisfaction from other pleasures. Then they tend to return with renewed interest to the pleasure of eating. Often they find the eating habit literally growing on them.

"Why not?" they say. It is a harmless habit, they think, as well as a familiar one. It is easy, requires no special effort. It is something to do when you are bored. It gives you a lift when you are unhappy, especially if you eat sugars and starches which are mild stimulants. It gives a reason for being with other people when you are lonely. It gives you something to talk about, think about, plan for, look forward to. Besides, it is necessary. You have to eat to live.

You do. But, little by little, as they grow older, many people begin to use food, not to maintain life, but as a substitute for living. For these unfortunates, eating becomes more than a body necessity. It becomes an obsession, something that many people do in spite of their will and against their own best interests.

Look around any restaurant at mealtime and you can pick out the overeaters, not only by their humpty-dumpty figures and the piled-up forkfuls of starches and sugars they are consuming. You can pick them out, also, by the discontented, rather petulant expressions on their faces. Overeaters are hungry, unsatisfied people. But often their basic hunger is not for food; it is for love, excitement, fun, adventure—all the good things of life that they fear are finished for them because they have passed the age of forty, fifty, sixty—whatever their age may be.

Such misguided souls thank heaven they can still enjoy a double fudge sundae with lots of whipped cream. They imagine there is nothing else left to enjoy; are not life and romance over? So they substitute the joy of eating for the joy of living. They shut the door forever on life and romance by making themselves into fat, unalluring, overstuffed human pincushions.

Once overeating has become a fixed habit, it is a very hard habit to break. Witness the endless procrastination, self-delusion, and alibis of the overeaters. Yes, they are overweight. They admit it, sadly inspecting triple chins, ruefully pinching "spare tires," apologetically panting for breath on a short flight of steps that should not give anybody trouble. They are overweight and they are going to do something about it. Going to diet. Tomorrow. Next week, when the holidays are over. Next year, when life has quieted down a bit and there are not so many of those ruinous luncheons, teas, and dinners that cannot be skipped.

Tomorrow does not come. The holidays are over but more holidays are just ahead. Life does not quiet down. At this point the alibis begin. It is not their fault, the overeaters decide. They are doing their best, but there are times when you simply must overeat.

Suppose a hostess presses a second portion of her famous lemon meringue pie "made especially for you." What are you going to do—refuse? Or suppose your out-of-town client loves fried chicken, candied sweet potatoes, popovers and waffles à la mode. What are you going to do when you take him (or her) to dinner at a famous Southern restaurant—order tea and toast? Or suppose you are eating alone some place where the food is wonderful but the portions are twice too big. Are you going to leave your dinner half-eaten, waste that good food when there are so many hungry people in the world?

That last alibi has always interested me. On the face of it, it seems plausible, although actually it is quite hard to see how eating food one does not need is going to benefit those who do need it. Overeaters are always plausible. They are as plausible as alcoholics.

However, their families and friends reason, it is up to them. If they prefer fudge to youth, health, beauty, adventure, that is their choice. They are adults; they must stand on their own feet; nobody is going to keep after them, begging them not to neglect themselves. Besides, perhaps their overweight is not due to overeating. Perhaps they cannot help being fat. Perhaps the fat is glandular.

It probably is *not*. Two percent of all overweight may be attributed to glandular causes. The other 98 percent is caused by nothing in the world but plain, ordinary overeating.

I believe that overeating, like alcoholism, is a malady. I believe that, like alcoholism, it is a symptom of personal maladjustment to life. Overeaters come to depend on the mental as well as the physical lift they get from their sugars and starches. It becomes as hard for them to pass a confectioner's as it is for confirmed alcoholics to pass a cocktail bar. And, like alcoholics, overeaters often abstain in public, and then yield to temptation on the sly.

That is why I have started a national organization similar to Alcoholics Anonymous for overeaters. That is why I hope that one day there will be a chapter of Eaters Anonymous in every city in the country. Nobody likes to face the fact that he cannot control his appetite. It is much easier to face it in a group of Eaters Anonymous who frankly admit that they, too, cannot take their food or leave it alone. Moreover, like A. A.'s the E. A.'s will find it a help in maintaining their own self-control to help others to establish and maintain theirs.

Such groups are united by a common bond—eating. Together they can help one another get free of their common bondage—overeating. By working out interesting and intelligent dietary regimes and giving one another moral support in sticking to them. By learning, together, to eat in a way they have never eaten before. Not negatively, to make life's sorrow bearable. But positively—creatively—to prolong and increase life's joy.

The common interest in food leads to the development of other group interests. There are far better ways of getting pleasure from the body than by stuffing it full of angel cake and devil's food. Dancing, walking, swimming, talking. Talking about food? Why not? Food is an exciting subject. Talking about overweight?

Again, why not? Of all the curses that destroy good looks and shorten and restrict life, overweight comes first.

"The smaller your waistline, the longer your life line." I have said this many times during many years; I shall never stop saying it; it can never be said too often. I offer it as a motto for Eaters Anonymous.

YOUR IDEAL WEIGHT

How much should you weigh? For your guidance, I am passing along to you the figures assembled by the Metropolitan Life Insurance Company in a study of thousands of insured men and women. These figures present a new conception of weight. Notice how small is the gain between the 15th and 30th years. Notice, also, that the chart does not go beyond the age of 30. This is as it should be. If you were normal and healthy at 30, what you weighed then is your ideal weight for the rest of your life.

Study the chart; find where you belong on it. The middle figures refer to medium-build, average men and women; the upper figures are for the small-boned, and the lower figures for the large, big-boned individuals. I, myself, am 6 feet, 3 inches, big-boned, much over 30 and I weigh 215 pounds. How much do you weigh? How much *should* you weigh?

REDUCING

If you are overweight, do not sigh, "It's my age." Age does not cause overweight. Do not sigh, "It's my glands." Glands do not cause overweight. Overweight is the result of overeating. The glands, however, do determine where the fat shall be deposited (see Your Glands, page 87). The first step toward normal weight for all types of obesity is correct diet. When you have freed your-

IDEAL WEIGHT CHART

MEN						WOMEN			
Ft In.	15 yr	20 yr	25 yr	30 yr	Ft In.	15 yr	20 yr	25 yr	30 yr
	92	101	105	109		90	95	97	100
4 11	102	112	117	121	4 8	100	105	108	111
	114	126	131	136		113	119	122	125
	94	103	107	111		91	96	99	102
5 0	104	114	119	123	4 9	101	107	110	113
	117	128	134	138		114	119	124	127
	96	105	109	113		92	98	101	104
5 1	107	117	121	125	4 10	102	109	112	115
	120	131	136	140		115	123	126	129
	99	108	112	115		94	100	103	105
5 2	110	120	124	128	4 11	104	111	114	117
	124	135	139	144		117	125	128	132
	102	111	115	118		96	103	104	107
5 3	113	123	128	131	5 0	107	114	116	119
	127	138	144	147		120	128	131	134
	95	114	119	122		99	105	107	110
5 4	117	127	132	135	5 1	110	117	119	122
	131	143	148	152		122	132	134	137
	109	118	123	125		102	108	111	113
5 5	121	131	136	139	5 2	113	120	123	125
	136	147	153	156		127	135	138	141
	113	122	126	129		104	111	113	116
5 6	125	135	140	143	5 3	116	123	126	129
	140	152	157	161		131	138	142	145

Ft	In.	15 yr	20 yr	25 yr	30 yr	Ft	In.	15 yr	20 yr	25 yr	30 yr
		116	125	130	132			108	113	116	119
5	7	129	139	144	147	5	4	120	126	129	132
		145	156	162	165			135	142	145	149
		120	129	133	136			112	117	120	123
5	8	133	143	148	151	5	5	124	130	133	136
		149	161	166	170			140	146	149	153
		123	132	137	141			115	121	123	126
5	9	137	147	152	156	5	6	128	134	137	140
		154	165	171	175			144	151	154	158
		128	136	141	145			119	124	127	130
5	10	142	151	157	161	5	7	132	138	141	144
		159	170	176	181			149	155	158	162
		132	141	146	150			122	127	131	133
5	11	147	156	162	167	5	8	136	141	145	148
		165	175	182	188			153	159	163	167
		137	145	151	156			126	131	134	136
6	0	152	161	168	173	5	9	140	145	149	151
		171	181	189	194			158	163	167	170
		141	150	157	161			131	134	137	140
6	1	157	166	174	179	5	10	145	149	152	155
		176	186	195	201			163	168	171	174
		146	154	161	167			135	139	140	143
6	2	162	171	179	185	5	11	150	154	156	159
		182	192	201	208			168	173	176	179
		150	159	166	172						
6	3	167	176	184	191						
		188	198	207	215						

self completely from the habit of overeating, if there is any glandular difficulty, consult a trained endocrinologist.

The first step in reducing is to make up your mind that you *want* to reduce. Look French pastry squarely in the eye. Say to yourself, "This will be a few moments in my mouth, a few hours in my stomach, and a lifetime on my hips—*and I do not want it.*"

The second step is to make up your mind that you will reduce for at least thirty days. Why? Because it has been wisely said that anything we do thirty times becomes a habit, and the only way to reduce is to form the *habit* of liking low-calorie foods. Forming of new food habits is just as important as actual weight; there should be not only a shrinkage of the stomach but a shrinkage of the desire for food. Remember that all of my People—Lady Mendl, Mrs. Ann Astaire, Grandma Reynolds, and the rest— have achieved long life and agelessness in the same way: by training their appetites. By making it their habit to eat intelligently. Spoiled appetites can be trained like spoiled children, but this takes time.

The third step is to make up your mind that you are not sorry for yourself. Are you a grownup? Now is the time to prove it by throwing away self-pity and putting self-respect in its place. You will be getting plenty to eat. In fact, if you follow the Live Longer Reducing Diet on page 301, you will not even feel hungry.

In supervising the diets of countless thousands of people, I have learned that it is important to keep the individual from feeling hungry. For that reason I have recommended fat-free yogurt (see page 261) fortified, a pint to a quart daily. Most people do not know that a quart of fat-free yogurt contains only about 150 calories and is definitely not fattening. Yogurt tastes so much better than milk, remains in the stomach a long time, and prevents "hunger pains." (These occur only when the stomach is empty.) In addition, the bacteria in yogurt are busily man-ufacturing in your intestinal tract the morale-building B vitamins which help keep your skin fresh and radiant, and make people say, "You're looking wonderful."

Also, in supervising reducing diets, I have learned the im-portance of a diet that is pleasing to the palate; it is generally agreed in modern obesity clinics that only such a diet can be con-sidered rational and scientific. Therefore I recommend that the protein intake be unusually high, that there be plenty of lean meat and all other first class proteins to keep the diet varied and flavorful and prevent a feeling of hardship. Moreover, protein foods can be called our best slenderizing foods. It was discovered by Dr. Lusk that protein has a specific dynamic action upon the glands of the body, especially the thyroid. Also, 100 calories of protein cause the body to increase its heat about 150 calories, and it is this extra heat which helps to burn that extra fat around your abdomen.

To help you further to prevent hunger pains while reducing, I suggest eating generous amounts of raw vegetables such as the finger salad (see page 279). Raw vegetables are not so completely digested as cooked vegetables, and they "stay with you" longer. Some raw vegetables contain only half the amount of calories when raw as they would when cooked. For the same reason, I suggest taking the whole of the fruit rather than fruit juices.

Naturally, all the different vitamins and minerals are neces-sary, but especially the vitamins of the B family. These vitamins, in connection with the mineral, calcium, will soon help you to overcome that unnatural craving for sweets. The food that gives you most of the vitamins of the B family with the least number of calories is powdered brewers' yeast; therefore it is wise to stir a tablespoon of it into all your drinks. Brewers' yeast, which is 46 percent protein, contains almost no fat. The more yeast you consume, the better you feel, and the more active you become. No more sodden sluggishness, disinclination to move a muscle. With yeast, you can regain the energy for normal activities and the sheer joy of being alive.

With a planned reducing diet such as this you can lose about 15 pounds a month. The longer you follow it, the more you will get into the habit of liking low-calorie foods, which will eventually solve your reducing problem permanently.

If you have 50 pounds or more to lose, do not be discouraged. Promise yourself that you will lose 5 pounds. When you have accomplished that (it is very easy), promise yourself to lose 5 more. By this time you will be pleased with yourself. You will look better and feel better; you will have new pride and self-esteem.

Promise yourself to lose 5 pounds more. Now your whole body will be in the swing of it. Before long you will experience one of life's great thrills—the feeling of victory as you look into your long mirror (your most honest friend) and see reflected the real You, which has been buried under rolls of unhealthy and unbeautiful fat. Every cell in your body will thank you. You can hold your head high. For somehow, with the layers of fat go feelings of inferiority and self-consciousness; emotional conflicts are sometimes lessened or eliminated entirely with the loss of disfiguring weight; with your new ability to control your diet, you gain confidence in your ability successfully to handle life's other problems.

I know a good husband who helped his wife reduce by buying her a beautiful and expensive dress in the size she wore when he fell in love with her. The dress hung in her wardrobe, waiting, a goal to be attained. The results were magical. Because the dress was beautiful? Because the husband cared that much? For both reasons, I think.

If you have pounds to lose, more power to you. Here are four points to remember. They will help you attain and maintain your ideal weight for the rest of your long life.

1. Protein foods keep the body firm. Eat them generously.

2. Learn to enjoy the natural flavor of vegetables with the minimum amounts of butter and mayonnaise. Yogurt can be made into a delicious salad dressing.

3. Break the habit of eating fancy desserts. No more gooey gobs of obesity.

4. Learn to enjoy coffee without cream and sugar, or drink café au lait, half coffee and half hot skim milk.

For the list of good things you can look forward to, see the Live Longer Reducing Diet on page 301.

SECTION *TWO*

YOUR GOOD LOOKS

VII. THE YOUTHFUL YOU

*I*N MY many years of lecturing I have found that there are two kinds of listeners. There are those who greet my Look Younger, Live Longer program with "Well—I'll try." Those are the people I know I shall never see or hear of again.

Then there are those listeners who say, "I'll do it." Those are the people whom I know I shall really be able to help, especially if they say, "I'll do it," confidently, but without do-or-die determination.

I have no liking for the spirit of do-or-die. I have seen too many tense, haggard, unhealthy and unhappy people driven by do-or-die spirit though worried days and sleepless nights. I believe that the secret of looking younger and living longer lies not so much in "willing" as in "wanting."

I call this Mrs. Astaire's secret because it is so well demonstrated by Mrs. Ann Astaire, who was referred to in society columns in London as "one of the most beautiful women of our time."

I first met her in the 1930's when her two famous children, Fred and Adele Astaire, were starring in *The Bandwagon*. A friend took me to the Astaires' New York apartment to tea. The conversation turned to health and youthfulness, whether it was possible to remain healthy and young by will power.

I said, "Not by will power. Those are the middle-aged men in bright neckties, the women who turn girlish in their fifties and go in for bright red shoes and hats. These people are trying to look young by force, as it were. I think being youthful is a matter of *wanting* to be youthful, steadily, all day, every day."

Mrs. Astaire smiled at me. "I am supposed to need glasses," she said. "I have a prescription for them. Do you think that I can avoid wearing glasses by wanting to, steadily enough?"

I told her that there were excellent eye exercises; that if she wanted to avoid glasses enough to exercise her eyes steadily—

"I'll do it," she said, with the note of quiet confidence that I like so much to hear.

I am introducing Ann Astaire to you for several reasons. One reason is that she is my very good friend. Another reason is that, although she is definitely one of my People, she is neither a celebrity, a career woman, nor a society leader. She is an unassuming, typically American woman, at home wherever she finds herself.

Born and raised in Omaha, Nebraska, she taught school for a time before her marriage. She was early left a widow with two small children who were soon to become a famous dancing team. Her children were the center of her life; wherever they were booked to perform, she went with them and made a home. She accomplished effortlessly the transition from Omaha to sophisticated New York. When her daughter Adele left the cast of *The Bandwagon* to marry the English nobleman, Lord Charles Cavendish, Ann Astaire made the transition from New York society to London society with equal ease and grace.

Her gentle, natural dignity amounts almost to nobility; she is internationally adored; the members of the British royal family are her friends. As her friend, I, myself, was welcomed into London's most brilliant and influential circles when I went there in the late 1930's to lecture on nutrition. In that way I was able to introduce to England the Hauser way of eating, which proved to be so helpful during the bitter, deprived war years that were to follow.

During the war, Ann Astaire took over the entire management of Lismore, Lord Cavendish's huge estate in Ireland, in order to free Lady Charles Cavendish for Red Cross work. Lismore Castle, already famous for its hospitality, now became equally famous for its cuisine; short-cooked vegetables and big bowls of crisp, tossed salads were a novelty, a seven-days' wonder. When food became very scarce in Ireland, fresh vegetables were still plentiful at Lismore Castle. Mrs. Astaire saw to the raising of them herself.

Nowadays, she lives in Beverly Hills where she can be near her son Fred and her grandchildren. She has the same quality that she had when I first met her—a quality not of youth but of youthfulness, of warm young dignity.

Her complexion is soft and unlined; she has healthy, shiny white hair highlighted with a bit of blue; her tall, slender figure is the envy of women in their twenties. She dresses simply, in quiet elegance, walks a great deal, gardens, enjoys her grandchildren. She is an active churchwoman, a believer in service to humanity and in the power of the mind to accomplish, little by little, the good it sets out to do.

She uses a lorgnette for theater programs and the telephone book, but she still does not need to wear glasses; she never had that first prescription filled. That first day I met her, she began making a part of her life not only the eye exercises I recommended, but the entire Hauser regime. With her characteristic quiet thoroughness, she has followed it ever since.

She eats intelligently; she has formed the habit of liking what is good for her, not because she must but because she wants to. She always undereats—again, not because she must but because she wants to. And she is always relaxed, for true relaxation comes from knowledge that you have yourself and your body under your own control, not because you must but because you want to have it that way.

And now perhaps you might like to go with me to Hollywood, where beauty and youthfulness are all-important, and let me introduce to you some actors and actresses who long ago accepted the Hauser regime with a confident "I'll do it." Hollywood stars have consulted me at all ages, but for those around forty there is no question of "Well—I'll try." These men and women really must do everything in their power to stay fit and vital.

The movie-going public worships youth and the movie camera exaggerates mercilessly every sign of age; it also adds pounds to the figure. Make-up is a great art but it will not conceal deep wrinkles and deep, dark lines around the eyes. Furthermore, movie stars must work long hours under grinding pressure, but their faces and bodies must never show the slightest sign of fatigue.

Let me introduce to you an actor who is the incarnation of masculine vitality. No one knows or wonders how old he is. It does not matter because he is ageless. Some years ago, when this actor first consulted me, he was a stage actor, thin, run-down, and wondering about his future. Nowadays I meet him frequently at Hollywood parties and when we meet he never fails to drink a toast to me in the form of a clear, fresh vegetable juice cocktail. He loses no opportunity to tell the world that I "knew him when" and started him on the road toward looking younger, living longer.

Let me introduce another slender, boyish actor who for the

past fifteen years has had a top box-office rating. No one is concerned with this man's age, either. It is his young exuberance that makes him so popular. Yet fifteen years ago, when he first consulted me, he was well on the way to becoming either a middle-aged "character" actor or no actor at all. He was well on the way to a paunch, a double chin, and a pair of jowls.

Here is the tall, regal actress with the husky voice and celebrated figure who, year after year, remains the epitome of what men want and women want to be. There is the short, plump ingénue whose contract specifies an ideal weight that will be the deciding factor in the continuance of her stardom. These actresses must remain ageless. But when they consulted me, some years ago, they believed they were "finished." They were shrinking panic-stricken from the merciless eye of the camera, running around and around in emotional circles trying to escape from the spectre called middle age.

To these men and women and to all others in all parts of the country, all walks of life, who are running away from their forties, I say the same thing:

Stop running. Youthfulness is not something under an auctioneer's hammer—going, *going*, GONE. Youthfulness is not retreating from you. It is you who are retreating from youthfulness, as fast as you can go, hurrying, hurrying. . . .

You have spent your life hurrying, getting born, raised, educated; earning a living, marrying, keeping up with the Joneses, having children, raising the children, educating them, marrying them off. It was necessary to hurry; there is a time limit for these things. No wonder you are breathless. No wonder your face and body show signs of weariness and neglect.

Now stop where you are. Say to yourself, "From now on there is going to be a change. A change of life."

Here it is. This is the change of life. The change of life is a change for the better. The hectic, hurrying, breathless years are over.

The change of life is nothing more nor less than a change of emphasis—less emphasis on others, more emphasis on yourself. It is a change of habits—controlling your body instead of letting your body control you. It is a change of pace. From now on you can stop hurrying. There is plenty of time.

Take your time. From now on your time belongs, not to your parents as it did in your youth; not to your children as it did in their youth; but to yourself. You can choose what you will do with it. You can spend all the time you want to on yourself.

Take your time. It is yours. And remember, you have one hundred years to live. It is much earlier than you think.

Until now, you have been changing, little by little, becoming a little gray or a little bald, a little wrinkled or a little puffy, a little too stout or a little too thin. "Too bad," you have said to yourself, "but nothing can be done about it. The women (or men) in my family always get gray or bald (or wrinkled or stout)."

Has it occurred to you that you may have become gray or bald *because you expected to?* Because when you looked in the mirror you were unconsciously watching to see yourself show signs of age, become more and more like some older member of your family whom you have been told, all your life, that you resemble?

Put this book down for a moment. Say to yourself, "I—this person sitting in this room, in this chair—I am a young person."

Say it aloud. Listen to your words. Repeat them. Accept your youth.

Now begin to visualize yourself as a young person. Recall

special events in your twenties and early thirties, special occasions when you were looking your best. The chances are that you have a favorite photograph or snapshot of yourself, taken at one of these times when you were on top of the world. Get it out now and look at it. Keep it where you can see it during the rest of the time you are reading this book. Why? Because you *are* that person, right now.

That is yourself you are looking at. However much you may have changed here and there, you still look like the young person in that picture. Your bones have not changed; neither have your muscles or the vital organs of your body. Inside the older-looking You which you see when you look in the mirror is the real You, the You in the picture. Certainly you have changed; everyone changes constantly. Why not decide right now to change, from this day forward, only for the better?

Within you the real You—the youthful You—is clamoring, "Let me out!" Resolve today to get rid of disguising lines, wrinkles, extra layers of fat, and set free the youthful You which lives inside you. Keep your favorite photograph steadily before your mind's eye. If you feel that you are that person, if you look for that person every time you pass a mirror, before long you will begin to see that young person in every mirror you pass.

VIII. REFUSE TO BE TIRED

FATIGUE

*T*HERE IS no *good* reason why people should tire more easily as they grow older. Constant fatigue is not normal, at any age. I believe that it is caused largely by dietary deficiencies, and extensive scientific experiments (both with animals and human volunteers) have shown this to be so.

At the famous Mayo Clinic, for example, several young nurses who volunteered for experimental studies deprived themselves of fresh vegetables and essential proteins such as milk, eggs, and meat. They put themselves on a diet of devitalized starches, cooked-to-death vegetables, white bread, white sugar, and gooey pastries. (A typical Old Ladies' Home diet!) Before long, these once-energetic and good-natured young women found themselves listless, jumpy, tense, and irritable enough to scratch out one another's eyes. And it ran in a vicious circle. The more tired they felt, the more they ate, in an effort to recapture their accustomed energy. But the more of their devitalized diet they ate, the more tired and listless they became.

Fatigue is a deadly enemy to our Look Younger, Live Longer program, one that we must wipe out, right from the start. Twenty years ago I learned, through my studies and experiments in nutrition, that people who ate natural foods such as whole wheat breads, whole grain cereals, whole sugar (brown), and blackstrap molasses were less likely to be plagued by fatigue. The tired ones were those who ate white breads, denatured and over-refined cereals, and white sugar.

Now it has been proved scientifically that these denatured foods have been robbed of the ever-important B *vitamins,* especially of B_1 (thiamin) which is necessary for boundless energy. An abundance of B vitamins is most important in outwitting fatigue; they provide the spark which releases energy from the foods we eat, much as a match furnishes the necessary spark for the wood in your fireplace or the gas in your kitchen range.

When I lecture I am constantly bombarded with questions about fatigue and how to prevent it. If you want to experience a quick pickup in energy (at any age) make your diet extremely rich in the B vitamins. You can do this by taking (daily) 3 or more heaping tablespoonfuls of powdered brewers' yeast in milk, or in fruit and vegetable juices.

Another type of fatigue in older people may be caused by inadequate amounts of protein foods. Proteins, as we know, contain the amino acids which manufacture the enzymes necessary for the production of energy. It is amazing how many older people still eat only one or two small portions of good protein foods daily, in spite of the fact that, more than any other foods, proteins are necessary for the muscles, glands, and energy production. Stop and check your protein intake for the last 48 hours, right now. (See page 348 for list of protein foods.) If you have eaten less than 60 grams a day, you can probably make that tired feeling disappear quickly by increasing your protein intake.

Still another (usually temporary) fatigue problem is caused by a decrease, or sudden drop, in the blood sugar. You can bring this on when you do not eat frequently enough. Many women have complained of this fatigue, which came on while they were so busy shopping for bargains that they forgot all about eating. You can prevent it by taking time to eat-for-energy. A stop at the soda fountain for a molasses milk shake will help pull you out of that slump.

Many of my students are strenuous people, busy, important, highly paid, indispensable. These men and women refuse to be tired. They cannot afford tension. Their lives require a full, steady flow of energy all day, every day.

For such men and women my Look Younger, Live Longer diet is a basic program. It is as much a part of their thinking as their political views or their professional vocabularies. When they think of food, it is in terms of lean, broiled or roasted meats; short-cooked vegetables; crisp salad bowls; eggs, cheese, fruit and milk. A quart of fortified milk or (preferably) yogurt, every day. Wheat germ, brewers' yeast, and blackstrap molasses are stocked on their household shelves as regularly as salt, herbs, and vinegar. So are tablets or capsules of such diet supplements as: fish-liver oil (vitamins A and D); ascorbic acid (vitamin C); calcium (such as dicalcium phosphate); and tablets containing iron salts and iodine.

These students of adequate nutrition have acquired the habit of eating correctly at mealtime and *between* meals. The latter are small snack-meals of fruit, cheese and crackers, fortified milk and fruit drinks, which ward off energy letdowns, irritability and nervous tension. The wise ones have learned by experience that there are just two secrets for living and working at a sustained pace, without strain, without overdoing, without knowing the meaning of fatigue. Their two secrets are: a balanced, vitamin- and mineral-rich diet, and the art of relaxation.

RELAXATION

Unless you are able to "let go" and relax, all the vitamins and minerals in the world will not give you a healthier, longer life. Our Look Younger, Live Longer program with its balanced, superbly nutritious diet will gradually establish for you a state of healthily balanced nerves to cope with life's ups and downs. Right now, you can learn "how to not waste energy" by learning the art of relaxing.

One of my friends, a delightful woman in her late sixties who has long enjoyed agelessness and who is a very busy and successful artist, summed up the point for me in a few brief sentences. She said, "Tension is age. Relaxation is youthfulness. Or you might put it another way: tension is ugliness, relaxation is beauty."

Who would be better qualified to define beauty than an artist? I think we can take her word for it. Relax. Remove the ugly tensions from your face and it will become tranquil, more harmonious and attractive, no matter what your age or features. Relax your body and it will serve you better, no matter what your age or figure. The men and women of all ages who are "naturally attractive" are not necessarily those whom Nature has endowed with beauty; they may be far from it. They are the ones you "like to be with," the people who never make you uneasy because they are so completely at ease themselves. Every man or woman who is truly great has learned this art of being at ease with himself and others; he is a normal, healthy, warm human being. I do not like to be in the presence of tense, twitchy individuals, regardless of their name or fame. To me, they seem immature; they have not learned the first law of successful living—to relax.

If I could make *you* relax and stay relaxed for the rest of your life just by talking about it to you, I would be the greatest teacher on earth. My hope is to do the next best thing: to get you excited enough about relaxing so that you will talk to yourself about it.

Ask yourself to relax. Ask yourself out loud. Listen to your words. Repeat them. Feel your face gradually change, your skin freshen and grow warm.

Do you know why this happens? It is because your energy flows where your attention is directed.

Frequently as we go along I suggest that you put this book aside for a few moments and talk to yourself. I ask you to repeat your words and listen to them. I do that because I want to direct your attention to yourself. The best way to attract your own attention is to talk to yourself. Out loud, if possible, but in any case using definitely formulated words and sentences.

Psychologists know this. Philosophers knew it before psychology was invented. Mystics know it; they tell us that prayer is merely a way of talking to our inner self. Doctors know it. They tell us that pain is Nature's way of calling our attention to an injured part of the body and directing to it the extra supply of blood needed for fighting infection and for healing.

All of us know from our own experience that there is another self inside us. Call it inner self, interbrain, central nervous system, unconscious mind; it has been called by all these names and many others. It controls important functions of our bodies, such as heart action, and directs the flow of our blood.

When I ask you, therefore, to ask yourself to relax, there is method in my madness. Notice that I say "ask" not "tell" yourself. You cannot successfully force yourself to do anything, least of all to relax. *Forcing only creates more tension.* You must really *want* to let go. Then, and only then, will you feel your muscles giving in and the warm tingle of envigorating blood flowing where your attention is directed.

In youth the blood stream is continuously pushing outward toward the surface of the body. There is no need to tell a healthy young person to relax and direct the flow of his blood stream to the muscles of his face, arms or legs. Nature is doing that for him. His skin glows, his eyes shine. He can play the piano or dance all night without feeling fatigue. Sleep is oblivion. A few hours of it and he is completely made over. In short, youth is relaxed all the time, though youth's relaxation is completely unconscious.

In maturity we relax by doing for ourselves, consciously, what Nature did for us in our youth. You can prove this basic fact to yourself right now.

Look at your face in the mirror. Now put this book aside and relax, relax your face, let go the tension. Talk to your face, yes, talk to it. In his excellent book, *Release from Nervous Tension*, Dr. David Harold Fink suggests using the words: "Relax . . . let go . . . relax . . . more . . . more . . . " You can use these or any other words that appeal to you.

Continue this for a minute or two. Close your eyes gently, not tightly. Let the different parts of your face relax. Talk to your tense forehead, your eyes. Cover your eyes gently with the palms of your hands and rest your elbows on your knees. Do not think— let go—breathe deeply—let a minute pass. Keep the eyes covered, make believe they are so relaxed and loose that they will fall out of their sockets (they will not). Let another minute pass, relax your mouth, your jaws. Let your head fall forward, limp, relaxed.

Now look at yourself in the mirror again. You will be surprised at the "facial rejuvenation" that has taken place. Even your eyes are brighter; you will see more clearly. All because you have *consciously* relaxed.

When you have learned to relax your entire body, at will, you will have learned the secret of agelessness. There are many methods and systems of relaxing, and all of them are worth exploring.

THE BODY SLANT

The simplest and most effective way I have found to relax the entire body is in the Body Slant position—with the head lower than the feet. I have taught this to thousands of men and women, and wherever body culture or beauty culture is practiced scientifically, much emphasis is placed upon its value.

There are many ways of achieving the Body Slant position. One is to go outdoors and lie head-downward on your cellar door, provided the weather is good and you have an old-fashioned sloping cellar door. Another way (if you are not too tall) is to lie on your ironing board, with one end of the board on the floor and the other end propped up with a low chair or footstool.

The best way is to get a board a foot and a half wide, and a little longer than yourself and, if possible, have a carpenter install it in a permanent place. The raised end should be *not more* than 12 or 15 inches high. If you have in the family an amateur carpenter with ingenuity and imagination, so much the better.

Many of my students in California have their Body Slant boards installed on the sundeck or in the yard. Indoors, some have had the board installed in a corner of the bedroom or on a wide window seat, and hinged so that one end can be raised and lowered. And many others simply keep the board upended behind a door when it is not in use. Have yours according to your individual preference and convenience, but by all means get the

Body Slant habit. It is the best way to relax at any age; after forty it is magic.

I find the Body Slant as effective as, and much simpler and safer than, the "head standing" method which was widely practiced about ten years ago by some of our outstanding people (including Lady Mendl, Anne Morgan, Ina Claire, Blanche Yurka, Greta Garbo and Elizabeth Arden). The Hindu who taught this remarkable exercise promised better looks and a longer life "because the constant downward pull of the muscles was reversed for a few minutes at least, and the blood forced into the glands and other vital centers of the body." While such a statement seems exaggerated today, the fact remains that when the feet are higher than the head, the pull of gravity on the body fluids is reversed.

In the Body Slant position, the spine straightens out and the back flattens itself. Muscles which ordinarily are somewhat tense, even in easy standing or sitting, are relaxed and at ease. The feet and legs, freed from their customary burden and the force of gravity, have a chance to release accumulated congestions in the blood stream and tissues, and thereby reduce the possibility of swollen limbs and strained blood vessels. Sagging abdominal muscles get a lift, and the blood flows more freely to the muscles of the chin, throat, and cheeks, maintaining their firmness. The complexion, hair, and scalp benefit from this increased blood circulation, and the brain also is rested and cleared.

Take the Body Slant for fifteen minutes, twice a day. Take it whenever you can—on arising, before retiring, or best of all, when you come home tired from work.

It takes time to learn to relax completely. Relaxation is a fine art. But relaxation is youthfulness. And you have time—remember? It is earlier than you think.

I know an important woman executive who has made it her daily habit to come home, undress, and take a short nap on the Body Slant board before dinner. Awakening, she consciously relaxes her eyes. Then she "hormonizes" (a 10 percent hormone cream is best) her face, neck, hands, and feet and lies in a tub filled with warm water, scented with bath oil. In the bath, she continues to relax—shoulder blades, calves, feet—and does the Stomach Lift ten or fifteen times.

Then, refreshed and rejuvenated, she is ready to dress for dinner and an evening of entertaining or being entertained. She is full of humor and vitality, her eyes are bright and sparkling and she needs no glasses—and she is past sixty years of age. She tells me that her before-dinner relaxation also assures her of deep, sound sleep.

EXERCISE—THE STOMACH LIFT

The Body Slant position is also the ideal one for practising the one and only setting-up exercise that you need do for the rest of your life. Yes, that is what I said—one setting-up exercise and only one. Here it is:

Lying completely relaxed in the Body Slant position, draw in your stomach as you count one. (Continue breathing naturally while doing this exercise.) Draw your stomach in and up, farther, on the count of two. On the count of three, you draw it in close to your spine, which is pressed flat against the board. Try to hold this position to the count of ten. Then relax, and repeat the exercise ten times.

I call this exercise the Stomach Lift. It was recommended to me by Sir Arbuthnot Lane, physician to George V of England. In the years when people were flocking to Munich to learn it at Dr. Bauer's famous clinic, it was called the *Bauchgymnastik* or "belly gymnastic." Anyone who has had training in the United States Armed Forces will recognize in this something of that old, familiar command to "suck in your guts!"

Do the Stomach Lift wherever you happen to be. Make a habit of it. On the beach, in the bathtub, when you are riding in an elevator, waiting for a bus, standing in line at a ticket window. Do it under the hair dryer, in a hotel lobby, sitting through a dull movie short.

Do the Stomach Lift for the rest of your long life, and save your waistline permanently. With it, you will save your posture, grace, self-confidence, and well-being. You will be saved from sagging shoulders, middle-age spread, "jelly belly," face and throat wrinkles, bulges and rigidity. Why? Because you will have a strong, permanent "muscular corset" supporting the center of all the vital processes of your body.

Within 30 to 60 days, you can have again a flat, firm stomach. (Remember that Grandma Reynolds flattened her "jelly belly" at the age of 85.)

Good health depends upon abdominal firmness; this region is the center of absorption, assimilation, and elimination. Energy and emotional health also depend upon it. Behind the stomach lies what is known as the "abdominal brain," a sympathetic nerve apparatus connected with all the other abdominal organs. It is not for nothing that we speak admiringly of a person who has "good guts," and when we say good guts, we mean firm guts.

And finally, you can do the Stomach Lift and be saved forever from the nagging voice of conscience telling you that you Must Do Exercises. If you insist, you can also do a "daily dozen," turn cartwheels, work out with a punching bag or rowing machine. I personally do not recommend strenuous exercise in the second part of life. But to Look Younger, Live Longer, you do not need it. You can be free of all that, for the rest of your long life. The Stomach Lift is one of the best of all gifts that I have to give you—the exercise to end all other setting-up exercises.

Master the Stomach Lift and, when you walk, you will keep your stomach flat without effort. Take long steps when you walk, feel the good, rewarding "pull" in the muscles of your legs and buttocks, feel your shoulders go up, your neck straighten to carry your head proudly. Imagine that you are a movie heroine walking down a long corridor toward the dramatic climax of the story, or a model on the runway at a fashion show. Or a dignitary crossing the platform of a huge amphitheatre to receive the decoration of the Legion of Honor.

If you want to have a "young" walk, follow an imaginary straight line, toes straight ahead, putting your feet down one in *front* of the other. Breathe rhythmically, exhaling deeply (the inhaling will take care of itself). If you have a dog or a grandchild, chase it. It is a good idea to get out of breath once a day, in any way that comes handy (except, of course, running up stairs). Walk where there are trees, if possible. Trees are breathing too, and there is a specific emanation from trees (an "air vitamin," so to speak) which is beneficial. Why else are sanatoriums built in the mountains and forests? Who would think of establishing a beauty farm or health resort anywhere except among trees?

SLEEP

Deep, sound sleep is a gift from heaven and if you have it, give thanks, for nothing is as rejuvenating as a good night's rest. I hope that you are not in the habit of taking barbiturates. Figures show that more than 6,000,000 people in the United States are unwise enough to shorten their lives by taking these so-called "sleeping pills." Do not worry about sleeping; the more you worry, the more sleepless you become. It is a vicious circle that you create for yourself.

I know one famous movie star who worried all day long about not sleeping at night. She not only worried about it, but talked about it endlessly. When night came, of course she could not sleep. I have no doubt that insomnia very often is caused by the *fear* of not sleeping. I have been able to help thousands (including the famous movie star) to acquire deep, sound sleep by teaching them to relax and by insisting on a diet rich in the foods which help to relax tense muscles and nerves. Many food factors contribute to relaxation, but the three most important ones appear to be calcium plus vitamin D, and vitamin B$_6$, one of the lesser-known members of the celebrated B family.

If you insist upon taking tablets to help you sleep, I suggest that you go to the nearest drugstore or health food store and buy yourself the biggest jar of calcium tablets containing Vitamin D. Any form of calcium can be used—calcium lactate, calcium gluconate, or dicalcium phosphate. Take two to four calcium tablets at bedtime, and drink a glassful of hot grapefruit juice sweetened by a bit of honey or molasses. Keep the calcium tablets on your bedside table and, if you feel the need, take more during the night. Ex-insomniacs around the globe have thanked me profusely for this incredibly simple method of regaining sound, natural sleep.

Even if you sleep well, get the habit of drinking a glassful of calcium-rich milk before retiring. The choice of fortified milk, yogurt or buttermilk depends on individual weight and preference. Remember that "soured" milks like yogurt or buttermilk supply calcium more completely. If these do not appeal to you, by all means drink "fortified milk"—half a cup of powdered *skim* milk beaten into a quart of ordinary milk. It adds delicious flavor to the milk and gives it twice the calcium content. Calcium, calcium, calcium—I cannot say it often enough—and I wish you would repeat it to yourself: calcium means rest, calcium means deep sleep, calcium means calmness and agelessness.

Vitamin B₆, the third sleep ingredient, is found in blackstrap molasses, but is not widespread in commonly used foods. It is removed from grains in the refining process and is not added to so-called "enriched" flours. Scientists who have studied this vitamin believe that our entire population suffers from mild B₆ deficiency; that our lack of it is the real cause of the jitters commonly ascribed to "this fast pace of living."

This vitamin appears to have a tremendously sedative effect on the nerves, and has even been used successfully (in massive doses) in treating cases of St. Vitus's dance and paralysis agitans, or palsy. That B₆ could bring about a relaxation where nervous and muscular tension is as great as in these diseases, indicates its great value to your nervous system and mine.

Here is our Look Younger, Live Longer nightcap, which combines the sleep-promoting food nutrients: a tall glass of milk (or buttermilk or yogurt). Into this, stir a heaping tablespoon of powdered skim milk, which adds more calcium and more flavor without adding any weight-producing calories. Last, stir into the milk one tablespoonful of blackstrap molasses for its vitamin B₆ benefits. You have one of the most delectable drinks you ever tasted, plus deep, sound sleep and happy dreams.

IX. DIET CAN MAKE YOU BEAUTIFUL

YOUR EYES

A WORLD of the future in which no one will need to wear glasses because mothers will eat a superior diet before children are born was predicted by Dr. Russell Wilder of the famous Mayo Clinic. This is indeed good news. What interests us even more in our Look Younger, Live Longer program is the fact that this famous doctor also says that if we apply our *present* knowledge of nutrition, we can delay the development of presbyopia, the kind of far-sightedness that often comes in middle life, and can even prevent the development of cataracts.

My first realization that we can actually starve or feed the eyes was a dramatic one. It came right after the first World War when thousands of peasants in Belgium developed a strange eye malady —nightblindness. Doctors were stumped, no medicine or treatment had any effect; it was wintertime and diets were therefore poor in fresh things.

Then spring came. The hungry peasants greedily ate the green buds and shoots which appeared in their gardens. Without drops or medicines, as if by magic, their nightblindness disappeared. This was a tremendous victory for nutrition. From it the whole world learned that *the eyes need vitamin A,* that fresh yellow and green vegetables rich in provitamin A can actually correct nightblindness.

We have since learned that foods like yellow butter and rich cream are even better sources of vitamin A; for best results eye doctors recommend high potency vitamin A fish-liver oil capsules. Not only does vitamin A correct and prevent nightblindness; it helps the tear ducts secrete their natural moisture, the best lotion in the world to keep the eyes naturally sparkling and attractive.

Decide, from today on, to feed your eyes for the rest of your long life. Every body requirement—every vitamin, every mineral, every amino acid—probably plays some part in the health of your eyes. Your best possible vision depends upon your blood stream's carrying to your eyes a consistent, steady supply of three vitamins in particular—vitamin A, vitamin B_2 (riboflavin) and vitamin C—and the amino acid, tryptophane.

Give your eyes at least 10,000 units of vitamin A daily as a safeguard against eyestrain, fatigue, and nightblindness, and also to keep them clear and bright. Vitamin A is manufactured in the liver by carotene, the yellow coloring matter found in carrots, apricots, and other yellow foods, and in all green foods such as parsley, spinach, and mustard greens; one generous serving will give you your eyes' daily requirement. Drink milk to supply riboflavin; citrus fruit juice to furnish vitamin C; eat eggs, cheese, and meat to ensure tryptophane.

One of my students, a musician in middle years, complained of an uncomfortable feeling of sandiness under her eyelids, which had become red and swollen. Tears accumulated in her eyes and they became bloodshot and strained. "It's my age," she sighed, looking for sympathy, making no effort to correct the condition. But exactly the same symptoms develop in a child, a youth, or anyone who lacks sufficient vitamin B_2 (riboflavin). A few weeks after she had eaten an adequate diet fortified with 3 milligrams of riboflavin taken with each meal, her eyes not only were normal but she had a new lease on life. She felt fifteen years younger.

Your eyes will serve you better after you have followed the Look Younger, Live Longer diet and have added the other special nutrients. I, myself, do not wear glasses, nor do many of my students; it is wonderful to behold the world through clear eyes. I am convinced that many who wear glasses could do without them but (and here is the catch) this requires time and effort. Rather than join the "throw away your glasses" school, therefore, I say:

Unless you are willing to feed your eyes, relax them, exercise the weakened eye muscles, for heaven's sake stop straining them. Get yourself the best glasses that money can buy. Be sure to go to a modern oculist, one who believes in and applies the magic of modern nutrition and who tests your eyes thoroughly. Well-fitted, good-looking glasses help you to feel and look years younger because they remove strain and tension in and around your eyes. Experiment with frames of all sizes and shapes. Big frames for big faces, small frames for small faces. Avoid anything fancy or tricky but do use colors; women, especially, should have several pairs of glasses in different colors and shapes.

Wear your glasses when you need them, but only when you absolutely need them. If you are far-sighted, as most people are after forty, take your glasses off when you go to the ballet or for a walk in the woods. Give your eye muscles every chance to relax, which they cannot do as long as they have glasses in front of them.

Even if you cannot do without them, take your glasses off from time to time during the day. Sitting at your desk, or wherever you happen to be, close your eyes, cup the palms of your

hands gently before them, shutting out all light, but being careful never to press on the eyeballs, and take a few deep breaths.
Let go mentally. Think *black*. Talk to yourself about black.
Shut out everything in the world except the idea of black—black
shadows, black velvet, black night.

This is the relaxation called "palming," which was introduced
some years ago by Dr. William H. Bates of New York City, and
is excellent for tense, tired eyes. Also, there are a few simple and
helpful eye exercises. I have seen weakened eye muscles so
strengthened and faulty vision so amazingly improved that I
am giving you six exercises; they were used successfully during
the last war. Hundreds of aviators were able to pass their strict
eye examinations after they learned to "palm" and to exercise
the six eye muscles. I hope you will do all of these. If you do only
one, let it be Number 5.

1. Turn your eyes up and down without moving your
head.

2. Turn your eyes from left to right as far as possible.

3. Look up and to the side through the corner of your left eye,
then down and to the side through the corner of your right eye.

4. Look up and to the side through the corner of your right
eye, then down and to the side through the corner of your left
eye.

5. Roll your eyes slowly, first toward the left, then toward the
right.

6. Sit out of doors, look at the tip of your nose, and then look
as far into the distance as possible.

Young, healthy eyes blink, constantly and unconsciously,
without nervousness, gently and quietly opening and closing.
Many older people, tense from head to foot, have tense eye muscles; they do not blink often enough; their eyes seem to stare.

Remember for the rest of your long life that we see *through* our eyes not *with* our eyes. Keep them relaxed. Decide, from today on, to blink consciously. When you walk, blink with each step you take. When you read, blink at each new line and prevent tension and blurring. Before long, you will again be blinking as you should do, unconsciously, and your eyes will look younger and serve you longer.

There is cheerful news about prevention of cataract. Cataract is neither a growth nor a film over the eyes but a clouding of the lenses so that vision becomes more and more foggy. Diabetic people seem especially predisposed to this. Cataracts can be developed in test animals by giving a diet lacking in the important vitamin B_2 (riboflavin). When large amounts of this vitamin are added to the diet, the condition is not cleared up but further progress can be stopped. Understand that this important member of the vitamin B family is no cure for cataract. It can, however, be called an important preventative. For this reason every one over forty whose vision is not good should make sure to obtain sufficient amounts of riboflavin. Brewers' yeast, yogurt or fresh milk fortified with powdered skim milk should be used daily.

If cataracts already have obscured your vision, do not live in fear and semiblindness. They can be removed surgically with a minimum of pain and danger. Find the best eye surgeon in your city, preferably one who specializes in cataracts. About four weeks before surgery, put yourself on the Look Younger, Live Longer diet on page 345 so that your own body defenses will be at top peak. You will be glad you did this.

If your vision is good, do not take it for granted. Feed your eyes. Relax them and exercise them. You will be well rewarded. Have your eyes checked regularly. They are an index to general health. Since eyes are so easily examined internally and externally, oculists can and will help us to find new ways to prevent illness and forestall age.

HEARING

Most of us are born with more acute hearing than we need. Nature is old-fashioned; she still starts us out in life with the kind of hearing which primitive man needed to keep alert (and alive) in the presence of stealthy, invisible dangers. But you and I do not live in caves; we meet few tigers or rattlesnakes. Many people retain acute hearing through long lives, but if, in the second half of life, hearing (especially for high tones) shades off a bit, this is nothing to worry about.

The wonder is that we retain hearing at all, under the constant barrage of roaring, squealing, grinding, clashing, screaming, banging, blaring sounds that assail us in our modern cities. We can be reasonably sure, however, if we follow our Look Younger, Live Longer diet program, of establishing and maintaining the sound nerves, balanced blood circulation, and vigorous general health necessary to keep a slight hearing loss from progressing further.

If you have a hearing loss serious enough to be a handicap, by all means do something about it to prevent further deterioration. There are at least 15,000,000 people in the United States who are hard of hearing. I say "at least" because that is the official figure of the American Hearing Society. In addition to these 15,000,000 who are known to be hard of hearing, there are probably 5,000,000 more who are hard of hearing and will not acknowledge it—people who are going through life always misunderstanding a little, always feeling a little misunderstood,

wasting valuable nervous, emotional, and creative energy trying to keep secret what everybody already knows.

If you are hard of hearing, face it with courage, patience, and
a wide-open mind. Courage, because impaired hearing is one of
the most difficult of all the handicaps to live with. Patience,
because there is no easy way, no miracle drug, no presto-chango
cure for impaired hearing. An open mind, because impaired
hearing, until recently the most neglected of all the handicaps,
is now gaining the widespread attention of top doctors, educators,
and electronic engineers. Today, whatever your type or degree
of hearing loss may be, you may be sure that otologists, audi-
ologists, speech and speech-reading experts, and hearing aid
manufacturers are working on your special problems. That is
why I urge you to face this handicap with an open mind and to
have endless curiosity about:

Diet in relation to hearing
Relaxation in relation to hearing
New medical techniques
Hearing aids
Auditory training

Diet is more important to you than you have ever before realized. Vitamins are indispensable requirements for good hearing.
This has been proved by experiments on animals, of which many
reports have been made. When the nerves on which hearing depends begin to degenerate, it may be due to vitamin deficiencies,
possibly extending back to early childhood. The myelin sheath
(nerve covering) is first affected by vitamin lack—especially that
of vitamin A and the B complex—and as time goes on the all-
important nerve junctions (ganglion cells) begin to disintegrate.
It is now thought that a vitamin B complex deficiency, if ex-

tended over a long period, will result in the disappearance of large numbers of these ganglion cells. Another discovery is that a deficiency of vitamin B₆ (pyridoxin) often results in lowered resistance to middle ear infection and in a dermatitis of the external ear.

But the B vitamins are not the only ones involved in the nutrition of the hearing organs. A vitamin E deficiency may be instrumental in bringing on a degeneration of the muscles of the ear as well as an abnormal thickening of the delicate bone structure. Vitamin A also is concerned in bone growth, and its inadequacy may be responsible for abnormal sizes and shapes of the bony parts of the ear. This overgrowth of bone, while not clearly understood, contributes to nerve degeneration. In both vitamin A and vitamin C deficiencies, the density of the bone is apt to be affected, and C is also concerned with nerve growth.

Those who are hard of hearing should daily include in their diet orange, grapefruit or lemon juice, yogurt, some form of cheese and a large salad of raw vegetables. I am convinced that if middle-aged people would eat well-balanced meals, many hearing difficulties might be prevented. The hard of hearing person should take brewers' yeast every day and supplement his diet with vitamin C tablets and calcium. Faithful attention to diet is your best safeguard against further deterioration of hearing; some of my students of long standing even report that through the years their hearing has improved.

Relaxation is of the utmost importance to you. Modern living is geared to auditory stimuli, to the sound of the doorbell, the telephone, the radio, the motor horn, the public address system. People with faulty hearing live in a constant state of tension which is reflected in the strained expression on their faces, the rigidity of their muscles—especially the muscles of the neck and back. They strain their eyes to compensate for their ears, and, since the nerves governing the eye muscles are centered at the back of the brain, they are likely to find their impairment literally as well as figuratively "a pain in the neck."

Protect yourself as much as possible from excessive noise of all kinds. Noise can be injurious; office and factory planners are just beginning to realize this and take measures to protect employees from all varities of what used to be termed "boilermakers' deafness." Do not let the radio blast your own (or your family's) ears. Turn it on only when you are going to sit and listen; adjust it to your hearing level. If this is too loud for the comfort of others in the room, have a radio mechanic attach a set of earphones to the instrument for your special use, or purchase one of the small, inexpensive radio sets with earphone attachment which are available everywhere.

If you are hard of hearing, face the fact that you need more rest than a normally hearing person, and see that you get it. Make relaxation your hobby. You will find deep-breathing exercises particularly valuable; I am told that hard of hearing people are likely to be shallow breathers, even to hold their breaths, unconsciously, in their effort to "pay attention." I am also told that they are likely to be so busy paying attention at the table that they swallow their food without chewing it. Relax—at meals, in conversation, everywhere.

Join a speech-reading class. If there is none in your town, write to the American Hearing Society for suggestions on how to get one started. Most hard of hearing people read lips unconsciously, whether they use hearing aids or not. To learn speech-reading and become skillful at it gives a great lift to the ego; classes are, in addition, a fine place to meet and relax with new friends who are in your same boat.

Have a checkup once a year with the best ear specialist in your community, either in his private office or in his hospital clinic. As recently as twenty years ago doctors could do very little to prevent or restore hearing loss. They removed ear wax, treated running ears, and dispensed sympathy. Today we can do much more.

Discuss with your doctor whatever new medical techniques you read or hear about; perhaps some of them may help you. The fenestration operation which has been developed by Dr. Julius Lempert in New York City is proving successful in a large percentage of carefully selected cases of otosclerosis. This incredibly delicate operation consists of making a new window into the inner ear and keeping this window open for the reception of sound. Dr. Arthur Kovacs, of Milwaukee, Wisconsin, and others report that in certain cases an artificial eardrum consisting of a moistened cotton pellet, placed on the promontory of the middle ear, creates an improvement of hearing.

Other treatments will be reported. As I have said, research in the field of hearing is steadily going forward. Follow this research. But do not be gullible. There was a time when the hard of hearing were preyed upon unmercifully by quacks, but that time has passed. Write to your State Medical Society for information. There is a vast difference between being gullible and having a hopeful point of view and an open mind.

Explore everything mechanical, also, by all means. If a test of your hearing on your doctor's audiometer shows a loss of 30 decibels (units of hearing) in the better ear, you need a hearing aid. If you are one of the lucky people who can get clear, undistorted hearing with an instrument (it depends on the type and degree of your impairment), get one tomorrow. Get it even if you have to beg or borrow the money. It will take ten years off your age. I have seen that happen repeatedly. A hearing aid can be one of the best Look Younger recipes I know of. A Live Longer recipe, too. I recently heard of an elderly gentleman who was so inspired by the possibilities of renewed living, with a hearing aid, that he exclaimed, "I want a *good* hearing aid, because I'm going to use it for a *long* time and I don't mind paying a lot of money for something I can use a long while." He was ninety-five years old.

A good way to keep an informed, open mind is through the American Hearing Society which has its headquarters in Washington, D. C., and 124 local chapters throughout the country. Through this organization you can learn how and where to get speech reading and speech training. You can explore the exciting new field of Auditory Training which holds out hope for better hearing with and without a hearing aid. Auditory Training centers are being established in many cities and research in this new field is going forward at a number of universities, including the University of Southern California where the Phipps Bone Conduction Unit was developed a few years ago. It is said that this instrument can stimulate the hearing organs and, even in cases where impairment is extensive, restore their function to some degree. A new method of improving the use of residual hearing by means of scientifically made phonograph recordings is also being widely and successfully experimented with.

To everyone, whether there is someone in your family who is hard of hearing, or you are yourself, I recommend that you read Frances Warfield's book, *Cotton in My Ears*. It is entertaining and amusing despite the seriousness of its subject. You will learn not only of the sufferings and pitfalls of the hard of hearing, but, most important of all, of how to live happily and successfully with impaired hearing.

For the rest of your long life, eat the foods which supply your blood stream with the nutrients necessary to the care and feeding of your ears. I believe that, thanks to medical science, the growing understanding of the importance of nutrition, and improvements in hearing aids and auditory training techniques, the handicap of impaired hearing can, within the next few decades, be largely overcome.

YOUR TEETH

"See your dentist before you are born," was the slogan of Dr. Mary Lohman, famous Chicago dental surgeon. Sounds silly? Not at all. If both your parents had the sound, healthy teeth that result from a calcium-rich diet, you undoubtedly inherited their beautifully healthy teeth. Congratulations, if you were so fortunate. And here is hoping that you also inherited their appetite for calcium-rich foods and kept the beautiful teeth which were your birthright.

Have you ever noticed the sparkling good teeth of foreigners who come to America, especially Italians and Scandinavians? And how, in a few years, they begin to have all sorts of cavities and tooth troubles, just as Americans do? If you have wondered *why*, here is the answer: our tooth decay problems are due to our calcium-poor and vitamin-poor diets and to our national overindulgence in corrosive sweets.

If you still have good, sound teeth, you need have no fear of losing them, whatever your age may be. Nutritious diet, not age, determines the health of your teeth. For all the years of your long life, feed them the four essentials for good, strong teeth: calcium, phosphorus, vitamin C and vitamin D, *every day*.

For calcium and phosphorus, drink fortified milk (or yogurt or buttermilk), and eat cheese. They put a gleam in your smile.

For vitamin C, eat citrus fruits, tomatoes, and fresh green peppers and drink plenty of fresh citrus juices. They will give you healthy pink gums instead of "pink toothbrush." (Bleeding gums are one of the first signs of vitamin C deficiency.)

For vitamin D, take fish-liver oil (in capsules if you like) daily. Vitamin D is the "sunshine vitamin" essential to your sunny smile. You probably are not getting much of it from your food and may rarely have time to get out into the sunshine where your skin can absorb it. It must therefore be supplemented, in your diet, in the form of fish-liver oil, *especially* during the winter months. As vitamin D is also essential to the complete utilization of calcium, it may well mean the difference between tooth soundness and decay or pyorrhea.

Americans are a nation of sweets-lovers, to the everlasting ruination of their teeth. Our overindulgence in candies, pastries, and heavily sweetened drinks paves the way for tooth troubles. The "cola" habit is an especially dangerous one. Long after the cola has disappeared down your throat, its sugar remains in the mouth insidiously eating away the enamel of your teeth. The chewing gum habit is another pernicious one, for the same reason.

If you are worrying about detrimental effects from fruits and fruit juices, do not let it deter you from enjoying tall glasses of fruit juice daily. Their natural sugars can be readily disposed of by rinsing your mouth, afterward, with just plain water.

Rhubarb juice makes a wonderful "beauty cocktail," not only good for the teeth but for the whole body. At Elizabeth Arden's beauty farm, it was extremely popular, served according to my recipe: fresh rhubarb juice mixed with fresh strawberry juice and honey. Try it and see for yourself. Also, rhubarb juice is delicious sweetened with just honey. If you have one of those wonderful vegetable juicers, by all means avail yourself of the health and beauty contained in fresh, tangy rhubarb juice.

With proper diet, your natural teeth can last you all of your long life. Remember that they are not only necessary to your good looks but to your good health. Teeth that are allowed to decay not only spoil your appearance; they make eating difficult, and infected teeth in turn can cause bodily infections which can destroy the nutritional benefits of the finest diet on earth.

DEAD TEETH

A report by Dr. Otto Meyer, of New York, to the American Geriatrics Society, states that: "Dental foci which are most frequently overlooked are small root fragments; devitalized teeth which in the X-ray appear normal but are nevertheless always infected; and infections of the jawbones. The tooth, periodontium, gingiva and socket form one unit, the 'odonton.' Infection of one part of the odonton invariably is followed by infection of other parts. It is therefore not sufficient to pull an infected tooth and leave the infected part of the jawbone. The bone infection must also be removed."

I myself have always considered dead teeth as enemy No. 1 in our Look Younger, Live Longer program. Seemingly minor infections can be carried to all parts of the body and cause trouble when we least expect it, especially in the heart and joints.

I shall never forget the near-chaos that one dead tooth caused the international celebrity, Lady Mendl. She had just flown over to America and was my guest in Beverly Hills, California, when she received a wire from Colonel McCormick in Chicago. The *Chicago Tribune* was holding its first American Fashion Show and Colonel McCormick wanted Lady Mendl to judge it. I urged Lady Mendl to go, for several reasons. For one, Chicago is the city of my greatest sorrow for it was there, at the Evangelical Deaconess Hospital, that I long ago was told to go home and die in peace. I didn't, thanks to the science of nutrition which I have practiced and taught ever since. I wanted to see Chicago again now, and I wanted Chicago to see Lady Mendl. This truly remarkable woman is a dear friend and faithful student of nutrition, and I am very proud of her.

We flew to Chicago and were greeted with pomp and splendor by Colonel McCormick. Batteries of photographers and reporters rushed to greet the fabulous Elsie de Wolfe Mendl. The *Chicago Tribune's* beautiful auditorium was packed with people. A special "throne" had been erected for Lady Mendl in the center of magnificent stage settings. The lights went on, the curtain rolled up, and standing before the footlights Lady Mendl was being presented to the audience as the internationally famous authority on style and beauty.

At this moment, the unforeseen happened; one of Lady Mendl's knees stiffened and refused to work. For one long minute we all stood helplessly, with bated breath. But, as usual, Elsie de Wolfe Mendl accomplished the impossible. Somehow, as though nothing at all were wrong, she walked proudly and erectly across the stage and climbed to her "throne." No one in that vast audience knew or suspected that for the next two and a half hours the fabulous Lady Mendl was in intense pain because of *one dead tooth*.

As soon as the show was over we flew back to Beverly Hills. Needless to say, that dead tooth was not just "pulled"; it was neatly and efficiently extracted, the socket scraped, and every possible trace of infection removed. And there was no further trouble in the knee.

If you have decayed and infected teeth I would recommend

that you go to the best dental surgeon in your vicinity (borrow the money if necessary) and have all sources of dental infection removed. Healthy teeth and jaws are a must in your Live Longer program. The modern dentist, with all the aids of medical science at his fingertips, works quickly and efficiently and with little or no pain.

To bring about quicker healing after tooth extractions, and prevent "dry socket" and other infections, put yourself on the special building diet outlined on page 345. Add maximum amounts of vitamins A and C, calcium, and vitamin D, and for the sake of the "inner man" drink a quart of fortified yogurt.

And when your dentist sends you a reminder to come in for a checkup, do not ignore it. He is doing you a favor and making it possible for you to have any small cavities quickly and inexpensively repaired, before they can cause serious trouble.

NEW WEAPONS AGAINST TOOTH DECAY

During recent years, dentists have been experimenting extensively with ways and means literally to "put themselves out of business," through the use of substances that, by impregnating the tooth enamel, would resist or prevent decay. For a while, fluorine was thought to be the answer. Then in 1946 a treatment said to be much more effective than fluorine was reported by Dr. Bernard Gottlieb (formerly of Vienna), of Waco, Texas.

Dr. Gottlieb's method is to seal up the microscopic canals which allow bacteria to get through the enamel of the tooth and into the soft dentin, where the greatest tooth decay occurs. He uses a solution of 40 percent zinc chloride, followed by a solution of 20 percent potassium ferrocyanide. When these two solutions meet, a chemical reaction takes place, producing a white salty compound which penetrates the entire length of the canals through the enamel to the dentin.

Since this treatment was reported, it has been improved and widely tested and is now being given by many good dentists in various parts of the United States. It is said that teeth so sealed are amazingly easy to keep clean. Hope is held that, with further development of this treatment, one good thorough sealing may be able to protect sound teeth permanently against decay.

A promising means of preventing dental decay, especially among adults, is the ammoniated dentifrice developed by the experimental laboratories of the University of Illinois. Back in 1934, the father-and-son team of Carl J. and Carl T. Grove, dental researchers in St. Paul, Minnesota, discovered that the saliva of persons seemingly immune to dental decay contained more than average ammonia, which dissolves the viscid coating that forms on teeth and breeds decay bacteria. Dr. Robert M. Stephan of the U.S. Public Health Service experimented with their discovery and found that the combined action of ammonia and urea (in saliva) counteracted the acid tendencies of the tooth's gluey coating and prevented decay.

With this knowledge, Dr. Robert G. Kesel and his research group at the University of Illinois concentrated on finding a suitable ammonia-containing substance to incorporate in a dentifrice. It proved to be dibasic ammonium phosphate. In combination with urea, it has the most effective action on the teeth's gluey coating and provides the quickest way to reduce the bacteria of decay (lactobacillus acidophilus). Today you can get this ammoniated dentifrice at any drugstore. For best protection, you should brush your teeth with it after every meal; in any case, do use it after breakfast and after the evening meal. Don't rinse it away when you brush your teeth; leave it in the mouth where it can mix with the saliva and continue to protect your teeth from bacteriological decay.

PORCELAIN CAPS

Sound teeth are not necessarily beautiful teeth. We have all seen people whose teeth were crooked and discolored, although apparently in a state of good health. Many of the sparkling Hollywood smiles that flash across the screen owe their enviable beauty to a dentist's cosmetic skill. Modern dentistry has discovered a safe and reasonably permanent way of capping teeth with fine porcelain or plastic.

If your teeth are discolored and uneven, you might consider the possibilities of having them capped. I have seen many people literally transformed, not only in appearance but personality as well, by having this done. But note that such teeth must be *alive*. (The old-fashioned, infection-breeding "pivot tooth" screwed into a dead root is fortunately now a thing of the past.) Modern tooth-capping takes time and is not without pain, but it is well worth the time and effort involved for the beauty and morale-lift obtained. The worst sufferer by far will be your pocketbook, for porcelain or plastic caps are both expensive and somewhat fragile, and with careless usage may be troublesome.

Our Hollywood beauties who have capped teeth play safe and carry a "spare" with them in their jewelry cases. Such spare caps are real jewels, often made on a platinum and gold base covered with a beautifully lifelike translucent porcelain.

ARTIFICIAL TEETH

Even if you have already lost some of your teeth, you need have no fearful qualms about wearing artificial teeth. They need not change your facial appearance for the worse. On the contrary, a good dentist can often improve upon Nature in this respect. He knows that your teeth should correspond to the shape of your face—narrow teeth for a narrow face, wide teeth for a wide face. He will give you artificial teeth of a bluish or yellowish white, selecting from dozens of available shades to match your own coloring. And for complete bridgework, he measures the distance from the tip of your nose to the tip of your chin and rechecks this measurement as the years go by. If this distance gives evidence of shortening, he can correct it by "opening" your "bite."

Do remember that although artificial teeth themselves do not need calcium and phosphorus and vitamins C and D your gums and the bony structure of your mouth need *all* of them—more and more and more—to keep your jaws from shrinking and to hold the dentures firmly in place.

If the diet is inadequate, the jawbones continue to lose minerals, and the most carefully designed dentures can then become loose and ill-fitting. Although your own diet is at fault, your dentist will probably be blamed. Then, too, with uncomfortable dentures, food is insufficiently chewed and is invariably followed by flatulence, gas pains, and other digestive disturbances. In contrast to this unhappy state, if an adequate diet is adhered to and the jaws maintained in healthy condition, one good set of dentures can fit well and work well indefinitely.

If you must have bridgework, by all means have the removable kind. When you have your teeth extracted, do not be without a substitute, even for one day. An immediate temporary replacement will not only keep up your morale, it also will keep your jaw from shrinking.

I am strongly in favor of the removal of dead teeth and all infection with them. And as strongly opposed to endeavoring to "save" dead teeth by the practice of filling root canals and thereby inviting infections. I could not be otherwise, since my life's work and teaching is a program of Look Younger, Live Longer.

The removal of dead teeth with the resultant removal of infection from the blood stream can add years to your life. Good bridgework and well-fitted, well-matched artificial teeth can take years off your looks and add them to your long life of health and happiness.

PYORRHEA

Another problem that has become widespread in our country, especially after the age of forty, is pyorrhea. This condition is basically one in which the jawbones become destroyed to such an extent that teeth cannot be held in place. That it largely results from inadequate diet is borne out by reports in the medical literature.

Dr. Martin Gumpert, of New York, in discussing changes that occur in teeth during the fifth decade of life, points out the importance of good diet and good dentistry in keeping teeth healthy. He states that control of the atrophy of the gums and the sockets containing the teeth, which causes the teeth to appear longer as the gums recede, "depends on the more or less healthy condition of the teeth."

Among native races on completely adequate diets, such as those studied by Sir Robert McCarrison, of England and the late Dr. Weston A. Price, of the United States, pyorrhea is unknown. A condition similar to pyorrhea can be produced in experimental-laboratory animals by giving them, over a long period, almost but not quite enough vitamin C. Since most diets are somewhat inadequate in all nutrients, rather than totally deficient in only one, deficiencies not only of vitamin C but also of calcium, protein, and vitamin D contribute to the appearance of pyorrhea in our civilized peoples.

In the light of all the scientific evidence, there can be little or no doubt but that pyorrhea is another manifestation of our national malnutrition. It is reassuring to know, however, that such teeth can usually be saved even after onset of the disease, if a completely adequate diet (such as that on page 249) is adhered to.

I believe that future generations, living on adequate diets, will continue to brush their teeth not to prevent decay—they will not have tooth decay—but because they like the idea of a clean mouth. In the meantime, remember that a balanced diet rich in large amounts of calcium and vitamins A, C and D can and will help you keep sound teeth for the rest of your long life.

YOUR HAIR

The war against gray hair and baldness is an exciting one in which, little by little, the enemies are being pushed back. For many years I have been following experiments in research laboratories all over the United States, some of which have shown remarkable results in restoring hair color and improving hair quantity on laboratory animals. I have also witnessed much human experimentation among my students, some of whom have achieved equally remarkable results.

I have no doubt but that one day the battle for hair that stays thick and healthy and retains its natural color will be won. And I firmly believe that it will be won in the same place in which the battle for longevity will be won—*in the field of nutrition.*

Right now, let us consider the available facts on the care and feeding of our hair. We all want healthy, long-lived hair. Some doctors say that the best way to get it is to have parents with long-lived hair. That is true enough; heredity does influence hair, just as it influences our entire physical make-up. The healthier our parents, the more healthy our own start in life.

I am equally convinced that eating habits—good or bad—as well as physical characteristics are handed down from father to son. Fortunately for the son, he can correct bad eating habits and thus hand down a healthier birthright to the next generation.

Anthropologists suggest that a good way to have good hair is to be Chinese. As a race, they have almost no baldness. Why? Well, for one thing, the Chinese live on foods rich in all the B vita-mins. Their diet is largely fish, soy beans, roots, herbs, unpol-ished rice, and short-cooked vegetables. The Irish people are an-other example. On their small island, the water they drink and many of the foods they grow are rich in iodine (as is seafood). A kind of sea greens, or moss, rich in vitamins, minerals, and iodine is used in a delicious blanc mange which is a favorite dessert. And to this day, you can see Irish men and women chewing this sea moss, either fresh or dried.

We owe our present knowledge of the importance of vitamins, minerals, and iodine in maintaining healthy hair to countless rats, guinea pigs, rabbits, dogs, and silver foxes; and to years of patient and careful research by scientists in experimental labo-ratories from coast to coast. All the way from the nutrition labora-tories of Good Housekeeping Institute in New York City to the University of Southern California College of Agriculture, studies of the relation of diet to hair go on.

From such studies we have learned that the growth of the hair and its pigmentation are regulated by the vitamin B family, plus iron and iodine. Some scientists who have done outstanding work on antigray hair problems have made the flat statement that *all* gray hair results from nutritional deficiencies.

Much publicity has been given to the antigray hair B vitamins, but the restoration of hair color is not a simple matter of swallowing a handful of vitamin B capsules and awaiting an overnight miracle. A lack of iron, copper, iodine, and some of the amino acids also contributes to untimely graying and a dwindling supply of hair.

In any case, while a diet rich in B vitamins plus iron and iodine can be instrumental in restoring natural color and stimulating regrowth of hair, such a diet must be maintained if the good results are to be maintained. In decades of observation, the only persons I have known to change their gray hair back to its natural color were those who had adhered to an unusually adequate diet for several years.

An interesting instance of this change of hair color occurred in a middle-aged woman whose hair had been completely white for some time. I lost track of her for four years. When I saw her again I was surprised to see that her hair had turned black, with just a wisp or two of white at the temples and the nape of the neck. Her explanation for the change disclosed an unusually intense application of the science of nutrition. Her reasons for this also were interesting: her parents had long been invalids, and their sufferings had instilled in her such fear of illness that the idea of building for herself the most perfect health possible became her chief aim in life.

As she explained to me, she had made a thorough study of the science of nutrition and for four years had adhered to a planned program. From commonly used foods, she had carefully selected only those which would make up an adequate diet. And daily and without fail, she had included in her diet ample quantities of the supplementary foods which provide the greatest amounts of the complete B vitamins: 3 heaping tablespoons of brewers' yeast; half a cup of wheat germ; 2 tablespoons of blackstrap molasses; and a quart of yogurt.

The change in her whole general health—energy, alertness and radiant well-being—was amazing, and she looked years younger than when last I had seen her. Ironically, though, she had preferred her white hair.

Three of the B vitamins—pantothenic acid, folic acid, and para-aminobenzoic acid—in particular are credited with restoring color to gray hair. In male animals (and some human males among my students), massive doses of the B vitamin, inositol, have caused a regrowth of hair on bald spots. Iodine is important for good circulation of the blood stream which feeds the scalp; a deficiency of iodine can slow down blood circulation to the point of causing slow growth and falling out of hair. A lack of iron results in an anemic blood stream.

From all of this it will be seen that a completely nutritional diet is essential to maintaining your crowning glory in a truly glorious condition. Lack of any essential nutrient detracts from the good obtainable from a semiadequate or inadequate diet.

All three antigray hair vitamins should be taken at the same time for proper assimilation, and they should be taken as food. Preferably uncooked food, since heat destroys folic acid. Brewers' yeast contains all three of the antigray hair vitamins. They are also produced in the digestive tract (especially folic acid and para-aminobenzoic acid) if you drink yogurt.

Incidentally, among the Bulgarians (whose national dish is

yogurt) I saw very little gray hair even on those who were over seventy.

The richest source of inositol is blackstrap molasses. It is also contained in brewers' yeast, wheat germ, and liver. Iodine is contained in sea greens and in fish, lobsters and other seafoods. Liver and wheat germ are good sources of iron, or it may be taken in the supplementary form of tablets such as ferrous mucate or ferrous sulfate. Sooner or later, vitamin manufacturers will include the three important "hair vitamins" in their capsules, and they should be recommended by all beauty salons and barber shops. Until that time comes, get your doctor to procure them for you.

For coffee lovers, the gray hair news is not good. There are indications that the American habit of consuming large quantities of coffee may be a causative factor in graying the hair. Laboratory animals at the University of Wisconsin developed almost every known symptom of multiple B vitamin deficiency, including rapidly graying hair, when coffee was added to their otherwise adequate diet. From these experiments it appeared that the coffee washed the soluble vitamins from the system. If you seriously wish to retain the natural color of your hair, I suggest that you try drinking some coffee substitute, preferably made with hot milk. If you feel that you cannot give up real coffee, try café au lait—half coffee and half hot milk.

One of the newer ideas about hair growth that is gaining momentum and deserves mention is that this body of ours, with great instinct for self-preservation, sends the important food nutrients to the vital, inner organs *first*. Only when there is a sufficient or extra supply of nutrient does it go for the outer adornment of the body, the hair, skin, nails, and teeth. Whether or not this proves to be so, it is a wise man or woman who sees to it that the entire body receives not just the minimum, but the *maximum* of all food nutrients as outlined in our Look Younger, Live Longer program. (See page 249.)

If you want to try to see whether your gray hair will return to its natural color, or an increasing baldness can be overcome, here are my suggestions: drink a quart of yogurt every day, and have a tablespoonful of brewers' yeast after each meal. Have half a cup of wheat germ for breakfast every day, and some blackstrap molasses (a tablespoonful) with it. Eat seafood and liver as often as possible. You can also take, in addition, tablets of powdered sea greens for extra iodine. And don't expect an overnight miracle; you will not get one. But in six months' time, with the *daily* inclusion of these food nutrients in your diet, you can reasonably expect evidence of darker and thicker hair.

One thing is certain: you cannot get new hair out of a bottle. Fortunes have been spent, and oceans of lotions have flowed in barber shops and beauty parlors, to no avail. There are as many theories about hair as there are worthless hair tonics. One doctor in Los Angeles came up with the theory that hair dies and loses its color because of "scalp tightness," and he believed that he had a sure-fire remedy for it. For awhile, he did a flourishing business injecting mineral oil under the scalp to create a "loose cushion." It sounded reasonable, and hundreds subjected themselves to this painful procedure. Even some of our movie stars, anxious to keep their hair in perfect condition, fell for this swindle. For swindle it proved to be, to the vast disappointment of everyone concerned. The mineral oil hardened under the scalp and formed unsightly lumps.

The only hair lotions I would mention—and that not so much

for their present value as because they indicate future trends—are the results of experiments by two well-known New York doctors.

Dr. John C. Rommell reports gratifying results in clearing up dandruff and preventing deterioration of hair by rubbing his experimental lotion into the scalp twice a day, *provided* the case of accompanying falling hair and dandruff is not one of long standing. Dr. Rommell made his hair lotion by putting thirty 5-grain tablets of sulfanilimide into a gallon of water and letting it stand for three weeks. It is, as he states, more in the nature of a preventative than a curative.

The other note of hope comes from the field of endocrinology. According to Dr. Max A. Goldzieher, both clinical and experimental observations indicate that estrogen (the female sex hormone) can be used effectively in combating loss of hair for both men and women. It has been demonstrated that estrogen applied to the scalp in the form of a hair lotion penetrates the skin and "materially decreases" the loss of hair. He adds that it "does not seem to influence hair growth; but stops or slows down encroaching baldness."

This estrogenic lotion is applied to the scalp by gentle rubbing with the fingertips, once or twice daily. In many cases, a decrease in the loss of hair has begun after two weeks of treatment, and progressive improvement (within four to six weeks) has reduced hair loss to "a fraction" of the pretreatment rate. Your doctor or neighborhood chemist can make up such a lotion, which surely is worth trying.

Whatever else you do, one of the best and most effective things you can apply to the scalp externally is a good, stiff hairbrush—or better still, a brush in each hand—vigorously used. The secret of good, healthy hair is good circulation of the blood stream—your "life" stream—carrying the above essential nutrients to all parts of the body.

An astonishing instance of the effect of circulation on hair growth was related to me by a well-known plastic surgeon in New York. He had to transplant skin under and above the eye of a man who had been injured in an accident. As the man was bald, the surgeon used smooth, hairless skin from his head. To the amazement of the doctor, a growth of normal hair sprouted out all around the man's eye. So incredible was this happening that the case was written up in the medical literature. A curious case, and one that points a curious question: is it possible that the hair cells never entirely die, and can be completely revitalized with revitalized circulation?

Whatever hair you have, whatever color it may be, be glad of it. Be good to it. Hang onto it with both hands. I mean that quite literally. Pull your hair, tug it, vigorously, once a day. Bend over (or take the Body Slant position), and pull your hair until you feel a warm, tingling flow of blood in your scalp. Keep your hair clean and free of dandruff. Brush briskly, to remove dust and dirt from the scalp and to stimulate circulation. Shampoo it frequently with a good neutral (not alkaline) shampoo.

I believe that both men and women would gladly pay a good price to have scalp massages and shampoos given in the Body Slant position. This position, by reversing the gravitational "pull" on the blood circulation, literally forces an invigorating sweep of the blood stream through the scalp. I predict that farseeing beauty parlors and barber shops will soon be giving such modern treatment, and will teach their clients to use the Body Slant position at home for health and beauty.

Never wear a tight hat. I suggest that you go even further, whether man or woman, and wear no hat at all except in severe weather or for the requirements of formal dress. Give your hair light and air, and give it a chance to breathe.

Now you are saying—what about hair dyes? And I say that to dye, or not to dye, is entirely an individual matter. For a man, unless he is an actor and hair dye is a necessity, it would be a terrible nuisance. (And so are toupees and hair pieces.) Man, in general, finds that gray hair adds a becoming flavor to his mature years.

For woman, it is another matter. A Frenchwoman dyes her hair not just when it is gray, but often when she does not happen to like its natural color. Coloring her hair can be as natural a cosmetic aid to a woman as making up her face and coloring her lips and fingernails. It can be fun. It can stimulate a new romance. And often, when a job depends on maintaining a youthful appearance, it can be a real necessity.

But make no mistake about it—hair dyeing is a fine art, and should be performed only by experts. Whatever you do, don't select either too blond or too black a shade as both can give you an unfortunately "hard" look. Do select, carefully, the shade which is most becoming and "softening" to your features and skin coloring.

The only reasons why a woman should not dye her hair are: if the hair is weak; then dyeing will do it no good. If the skin is thin and delicate; the dyeing will take away from the complexion's softness, whereas natural gray hair will enhance it. If price is a consideration, do not dye unless you can afford an expert's prices. Remember that once dyed, hair must be kept meticulously retouched, at regular intervals. Do not attempt to "save money" with botchy, self-done dye work; you will have saved your purse at the expense of your appearance and the health of your hair.

All other reasons against a woman's dyeing her hair belong to the Dark Ages.

In conclusion, it is my opinion that while color may be a good and desirable thing, the really important and desirable thing is that hair be alive and shining. You can achieve that only if you keep the entire body in glowing health through sound nutrition.

YOUR SKIN

Since the days when it was not only modern and unique but revolutionary to do so, I have preached the gospel of "Eat and Grow Beautiful." *Vogue*, America's magazine for sophisticates, was first to print my diets, and the response of American women was tremendous. Those who could afford to do so, flocked to Elizabeth Arden's beauty farm where my diets were served. When I realized what an immense hunger for beauty existed, I promptly wrote my book *Eat and Grow Beautiful*, making my diet available to all women. So enthusiastically was this received that one might almost think women would rather be beautiful than healthy. Fortunately, my way of eating brings health as well as beauty.

It is my hope that such beauty farms, health resorts, and clubs will spring up all over the United States for men and women of average income. There should be thousands of such places where, for moderate sums, everyone can go and relax in the sun and be served delicious, healthful meals; where they can drink fresh vegetable and fruit juices to their hearts' content; and fortified milk with its rich protein to strengthen tired, flabby bodies and faces. And where the Body Slant is practiced three times a day; weary bodies massaged and oiled with organic oils and lotions; and the dead dry skin of face and body removed daily with simple spatulas as was done by the Greeks in their solariums, centuries ago.

Like all other parts of the body, your facial skin is made up of proteins. The surface skin, its tissues, and all its tiny muscles can be kept youthful only by protein foods which supply all the essential amino acids. With inadequate supplies of proteins and the amino acids, the tissue begins to sag, causing wrinkles to appear. Therefore, to prevent and to halt undesirable wrinkling, you must see to it that your daily diet contains ample amounts of tissue- and muscle-building proteins.

To counteract sagging muscles, also, think in terms of proteins. Never forget that facial muscles are living elastic tissue and that they can be nourished and built up from the inside with a good diet especially high in first class proteins such as meats, cheese, eggs, milk, and legumes.

Vitamins also are important to the rebuilding of tissues and muscles, and prevention of wrinkling. Between the protein cells of the skin is a "cementing" substance, collagen, which depends upon adequate supplies of vitamin C for its elasticity. The B vitamin, pantothenic acid, also is invaluable to an unwrinkled skin. When laboratory animals are fed a diet adequate in all respects except for pantothenic acid, even the *young* animals develop the grayed and wrinkled aspects of advanced old age.

It is not by accident that some persons of sixty or seventy have skin which is still firm, smooth and attractive. Would it surprise you to learn that these envied ones prefer cheese and fruits for dessert, and never stuff themselves with devitalized candies and pastries? They have achieved that envied surface through what they fed the inner man!

As the complexion grows older it tends to become dry, perhaps rough. Dryness and roughness indicate vitamin A deficiency.

This is the vitamin, you remember, which is manufactured in the liver from the coloring matter found in carrots, apricots, cantaloupe, and other yellow foods, and in leafy green foods such as parsley, spinach, beet and turnip tops, mustard greens. You remember, also, that excess vitamin A is never wasted, but is stored in the body fat. Eat plenty of green and yellow vegetables, drink a glass of fresh vegetable juice every day, and know that vitamin A will be stored in the fat just beneath the surface of your skin, counteracting any tendency to dryness and roughness, giving your complexion the warm, natural glow that you want it to have for the rest of your long life.

All the vitamins of the B family, also, are important in keeping your skin youthful. In fact, so important are they that most people notice improvement in skin texture and aliveness within a week after adding brewers' yeast to the daily diet. Vitamin B_1 keeps skin rosy and well nourished by keeping blood circulation normal, and is especially important to "palefaces." A deficiency of vitamin B_2 (riboflavin) can be the cause of that ugly pigmentation on face and hands. This condition, generally associated with "age," diminishes gradually when riboflavin is liberally supplied. Excessively oily skin, cracked skin, and small deposits of fat also can sometimes be traced to riboflavin deficiency; youth and beautywise, this is an indispensable member of the B family and its richest sources are liver, brewers' yeast, wheat germ, and fortified milk, yogurt, or buttermilk.

THOSE DEEP, DARK CIRCLES

Have you got deep, dark circles around your eyes? Why? Because you are feeling older? That could be the reason.

But suppose it is the other way around. Suppose you are feeling older because when you look at your eyes in the mirror you see deep, dark circles around them.

The tissues around your eyes are thinner than the tissues of the rest of your face. Pinch the skin under your eyes gently, then pinch your cheek; you see what a difference there is. Where skin is thin, blood flows close beneath its surface and the color of the blood shows through. Rich, bright-red blood makes a clear, rosy complexion. Darkened, bluish blood makes the whole face look pale; around the eyes, where the blood stream is just under the surface, it paints the skin bluish. When you see dark circles, then, know that your blood stream, instead of being bright red and full of oxygen and nutrients, is dark red with an overbalance of carbon dioxide and waste products.

Know also that some foods, when digested, liberate more carbon dioxide gas and acid products than other foods do, and tend, therefore, to darken the blood. Such foods are cereals, breads, flour pastes and pastry—all foods, in fact, that are rich in starch. Since proteins—meats, peas, beans, cheese, and eggs—break down into acids during digestion they, also, tend to darken the blood.

You need starch, of course. You need protein, definitely. But balance these with more antacid foods than you have been getting. Eat more and more fruit, especially citrus fruit. More and more leafy and brilliantly yellow vegetables. Fortify your blood stream and make it a richer and brighter red. Drink two or three glasses of carrot and parsley juice each day. Instead of eating candies and cookies, squeeze a glassful of fresh orange juice and drink a toast to the disappearance of your deep, dark circles.

MAKE FRIENDS WITH YOUR FACE

There are exactly fifty-five muscles in your face; with these muscles you express all your feelings. The muscles are "wired" with nerves and these nerves are connected with your brain and are related, therefore, to every part of your body. Everything you think, everything you do, everything you eat—pleasant or unpleasant, healthy or unhealthy—eventually shows up in your face. Each habit, good or bad, brings into play certain sets of the fifty-five muscles and produces folds, lines and wrinkles. It would be impossible to make a wrinkle all at once; you must tense and pull muscles fiercely every day for years before wrinkles become noticeable, conspicuous, and permanent.

A famous plastic surgeon says that lines and wrinkles are an index to personality. Stubborn, self-willed people who are set in their ways press their lips together tightly until they have deep wrinkles on the upper lip. The earliest wrinkles appear around the eyes; these are not necessarily due to age; they may be mirth or laughing lines. Wrinkles between the eyes, especially if they are deep, indicate excessive determination; they are often found in homemakers who are overly efficient or in people who drive themselves in some other way.

It is the daily overuse of the same facial muscles that forms lines and wrinkles in the skin. This explains why certain occupations and professions produce the same kinds of lines and wrinkles. Have you noticed that many speakers, lawyers, and actors have deep lines in the middle of the cheek, going all the way down to the chin? A forceful business executive often has a few wrinkles directly under his nose. Dressmakers, secretaries, and others whose jobs necessitate pushing the chin down often have an extra roll or double chin. People who have been ill or have suffered a great deal frequently have very fine wrinkles all over the face. Unbalanced reducing diets also can cause lines and wrinkles. By no means *all* lines are caused by age. By no means are all lines undesirable. Some lines are desirable. How often you see a person who has been plain become increasingly attractive with age. And how often you see a mature person with a baby-smooth face, and sense that this is a person who is superficial and wanting in feeling.

Do not worry about character lines and fine wrinkles. Just be sure that they are in the right places and that they have an upward, not a downward, slant.

If the lines of your face go downward, it may be for no other reason than the fact that for years you have been looking in the mirror only for the purpose of seeing what was wrong with your face. You may have confronted it each day as a burden and a responsibility, saying to it, in effect, "All right. I will wash you. I will shave you or put on cold cream and powder. I will make the best of you. But I do not think much of you. You are getting older every day of your life."

When you are away from your mirror, washed, groomed or made up, and someone greets you with "How well you are looking," your face flushes and smiles with pleasure. All its lines immediately turn upward. But you do not see that. You seldom have the pleasure of seeing your face when it is happy and animated, looking its youngest and best.

Look at yourself in the mirror. Now. Pretend, for a moment, that you have been invited to try out for a part in a play. You have been given this line to read: "You are no friend of mine—I don't like you."

Say the line aloud. You are trying out for a part in a play, remember. Repeat your line. Mean it. Give it full dramatic value;

you really want a part in this play. Look at your face in the mirror as you deliver your line. Watch the pull of your facial muscles. Which way do they go? Downward, of course. It is impossible to speak that line and mean it (it is impossible even to think the line and mean it) without pulling your facial muscles down.

Now, suppose that you have read your line superlatively well. You have dramatic ability. You are given a second tryout and this time your line is: "We are friends—I like you very much."

Give that line its full dramatic value. You are good, remember; you are a runner-up in the competition, almost certain of getting a part in the play. Rehearse your line. Give it everything you have. Watch yourself in the mirror. Do you see how the muscles of your face go upward?

From now on, when you look in the mirror, examine your face to see, not how old, but how young it looks. This is not vanity; I do not suggest that you spend your time admiring yourself. I do suggest that you make it your habit to look at yourself positively, constructively. That you look at your face as you would look at a friend, with tolerance, interest and affectionate regard.

YOUTHFULNESS FROM THE OUTSIDE

Keeping the complexion youthful is an internal-external affair. When you have made it your habit to eat so that your blood stream contains all the elements necessary to nourish your skin, you insure youthfulness from the inside. Every time you bend over, every time you run for the bus, every time you spend fifteen minutes in the Body Slant position—every time, in short, that you do anything to send a fresh supply of rich, red blood to your face, you are giving yourself a beauty treatment.

Next come regular and effective habits of caring for the skin from the outside. For women, this becomes increasingly important with age. The great outside enemy of youthful skin is dryness; keep this uppermost in mind. Protect your face against sunburn and windburn. Do not live in rooms that are overheated. Get out of doors in damp weather. Remember that English women have naturally beautiful complexions and that they probably have the moisture and freshness of air in Great Britain to thank for it.

Use super-fatted soaps, cleansing creams, lotions and foundations that contain a balanced combination of vegetable, animal and mineral oils made especially for dry skin. Dr. K. K. Jones and D. E. Murray from Northwestern University made an amazing discovery which has been ignored by most manufacturers of cosmetics: that cholesterol (the waxy substance which is so damaging to the arteries on the inside) when added to petrolatum and the cheaper mineral oils, increases the cleansing efficacy of creams and lotions by 1,200 percent. I consider this discovery, and the addition of estrogen (the female sex hormone) to complexion cream, the two most helpful and interesting developments in the entire cosmetic field. It is my deep hope that all cosmetic manufacturers will embody and apply this newer knowledge and thus put healthier and younger-looking complexions within reach of all women in the second half of life.

As to estrogen, the knowledge that it can freshen dry skin from the outside comes from Vienna, where it was discovered that after middle age the ovaries secrete fewer hormones and that this causes the complexion to lose its tone. Since these female hormones have become stabilized, estrogen-containing ointment has been produced which, I am told by authorities—among them the eminent New York endocrinologist, Dr. Max A. Goldzieher—can result in pronounced regeneration of aging skin.

Dr. Goldzieher points out that the female sex hormone is

needed not only for the function and maintenance of the genital organs and secondary sex characteristics, but plays a role in the metabolism of most tissues of the body, especially the skin, which is particularly in need of estrogenic stimulation. Estrogen, he says, is the one hormone singularly well fitted for cosmetic administration, since it is readily absorbed when applied externally in a suitable ointment base. Such ointment can be of value to women who have reached and passed menopause, but is not limited to menopausal women; the skin may need extra estrogen at any age. He recommends, in fact, the early use of estrogen cream as a method of delaying and perhaps preventing skin changes that are noted in older women.

I recommend that all women past forty begin "hormonizing" their complexions every night with a cholestrin-base ointment containing 10,000 units of estrogen per ounce. This, in combination with high-vitamin, mineral, and protein foods, is today the best method known of permanently freshening tired faces and preventing further premature aging.

Talk over your complexion problem with a reliable beauty specialist. There are excellent ones in all the larger cities. Do not be the naive woman who tries everything and sticks to nothing, but watch out for all methods, be they old or new, which promote the circulation of blood in the face and prevent a "hanging face" and dry skin. A mildly stimulating unguent containing a small amount of balsam of Peru applied to the face and neck is amazingly effective for the face and sagging throat muscles. Remember that all beauty treatments are more effective when taken in the Body Slant position. Already some of the New York beauty salons apply this principle. On the Arden beauty farm each room is equipped with a slanting couch; at Richard Hudnut's, facial treatments are given on luxurious couches with the head lower than the feet. Beautymasters of Beverly Hills, California, have incorporated the Body Slant in their inside-outside beauty plan, insisting that all facial treatments, circulatory treatments for the eyes, and scalp treatments be taken in this position. Beauty-masters are trained in the science of nutrition for building up or reducing, but their great specialty is "youthifying" the mature woman by every possible means. These trained specialists can be of immense value in our Look Younger program and can be found in many large cities. See if Beautymasters is listed in your telephone directory; if not, write to them directly in Beverly Hills, California, for information.

X. OTHER AIDS TO BEAUTY

PLASTIC SURGERY

*T*HE LAST time I lectured in Denver, I saw Jane Kent in my audience. Miss Kent is a Hauser student of long standing; she is one of the highest-salaried business women west of the Mississippi. She seemed to be listening intently.

Afterwards, she said to me, "I didn't hear a word you said after your opening sentence about how everybody can live to be one hundred years old. I began thinking about houses."

"Houses?"

She nodded. "Suppose you take a house on a short or an indefinite lease. It's not just what you want, but who cares? Suppose, however, that you take a house on a hundred-year lease. That's different. If it's not what you want, you do something about it."

She looked me squarely in the eye. "I've had a disfiguring nose all my life. I've succeeded in spite of it. But I think I'll be a lot happier and more successful if I have it remodeled. Anyhow, if I'm going to live to be one hundred, I've got time to find out. How do I go about finding a good plastic surgeon in Denver?"

The way to find a good plastic surgeon is the same, wherever you live. Write to the State Medical Society at your state's capitol and ask for the names of at least three doctors who are licensed to do plastic surgery in your vicinity. Find out all you can about these doctors. Find out whether they have hospital affiliations. Consult the Cumulative Index of Medicine in your local library to find out if they have contributed to medical journals. Consult the doctors themselves and ask, if possible, to see some of their work. Often you will find that these doctors' nurses have had plastic surgery performed and do not hesitate to show the corrections.

In other words, if you are considering plastic surgery, find a first-rate doctor, an artist in his profession. Remember that first-rate doctors never advertise. Remember, also, that first-rate plastic surgery may come high but is cheap at any price, whereas second-rate work is ruinous, at any price.

Among the great favorites of stage and screen are many who have had such surgical reconstruction of their faces, or of specific features. One of the most popular Hollywood beauties recently spent one month having her entire face and neck reconstructed by the best and most modern plastic surgeon obtainable. Plastic surgery is not at all what most people think it; the horror tales that get around are simply examples of ruinous, second-rate work. Contrary to popular supposition, the "two weeks in hospital with horrible suffering" does not exist in good plastic surgery, which is largely performed in meticulously maintained private operating rooms, not general hospitals. Nose operations, which are very popular and quite common, are achieved in an amazingly short time, and the patient returns home to apply ice packs during the short healing period.

Puffy bags under the eyes can be discordant in an otherwise-harmonious face. They are usually caused by deposits of fat globules; they can be permanently removed, without scarring, by a good plastic surgeon. I recently watched such an operation in Paris. The surgeon, famous for his artistry and skill, performed the operation on his wife. Using a tiny knife that looked very much like a fountain pen, he made an incision in the fine laugh-lines under the lower eyelid and removed the accumulated bag of fat globules. About eight stitches closed the incision, and three days later, when the stitches were removed, there was only a very fine line (easily covered with make-up) for about four weeks. Today, there is no sign of a scar or other indication that the oper-ation was performed; the improvement in the woman's appear-ance is astonishing, and she is the best possible "ad" for her surgeon-husband's work.

I was very interested to learn that Lady Mendl had had this operation performed many years ago by the famous Dr. Gillis in London. Lady Mendl has always been glad that she did so; she says that she hated puffy eyes, did not feel that they belonged to her, and saw no reason why she should put up with them unnec-essarily.

If your face has served you well for all these years and is not disproportionate (even if it is not the "ideal" oval type), forget about plastic surgery. But (and this is an important "but") if your nose outbalances your other features, or puffy bags and badly prolapsed cheeks are making you unhappy, or a bad neck or other defect has caused you anguish all your life, then, by all means, have it corrected. Then, I say, let beautifully changed features be a part of the change in your life; a part of your more beautiful and harmonious long life. Especially, have plastic sur-gery if your livelihood depends upon putting your best face for-ward. Plastic surgery has made truly amazing progress since World War II, and many, many surgeons learned the fine artistry of reconstructing battle-shattered bodies and faces.

I believe in plastic surgery. I have seen mature men's lives transformed by simple reshaping of a disfiguring feature. I have seen mature women's morale and earning capacity restored by a face lift, and the psychological effect is often as important as the actual lift. I look forward to the time when the remedying of bodily blemishes and deformities, at all ages, by expert plastic surgeons will be taken as a matter of course, much the same as going to the dentist to have teeth repaired, replaced, or capped. I hope and believe that plastic surgery will soon become a well-regulated therapy, free from hush-hush and free from the unscrupulous practitioners who thrive in any field that is clouded by moral prejudice and social disapproval.

Face peeling is another rejuvenating technique which is good when well used, dangerous when misused. I know of many men and women who have had themselves "skinned" with dangerous deep peels. When the new skin appeared, all pink and pretty, they realized to their sorrow that they did not like it; their hair, eyes, and the rest of their bodies did not harmonize with their pink-and-white faces; the skin looked strange and unhealthy, the acids had also destroyed some of the "oil cells" and the face had to be powdered heavily. Yet I do not rule out face peeling. At times I recommend a mild skin peel to relieve surface tension. But deep peels should never be resorted to unless it is for the removal of deep scar tissue; no peeling of any kind should be done by any except a first-rate physician.

SUPERFLUOUS HAIR AND MOLES

As the years go by, superfluous hair on the face becomes a real problem for many women. Moles also appear, sometimes covered with hair. In some countries, France, for example, facial hair is not objected to; I understand that there is even a province in Japan where a woman's beauty is judged by the length of her mustache. In this country, however, hair on a woman's upper lip and chin seems unfeminine and unbeautiful and may be the cause of unnecessary mental distress.

A thorough physical checkup is in order in all such cases, with a check on various glandular functions, including a basal metabolism test. If endocrine deficiencies are present, they should be treated. Then, for vanity's sake and for the sake of one's family and friends, have the hair removed. In mild cases depilatory wax is best; this removes hair readily and discourages regrowth. There is no truth in the old wives' tale that for every hair you pull out, two new ones appear. For permanent removal the only safe method is electrolysis, which has been used by dermatologists since 1875. This treatment should be given by a trained technician. For such sensitive areas as the face, use of a single needle rather than multiple needles is recommended. Strong hairs are difficult to destroy; often they must be removed more than once. But with patience on the part of the subject and skill on the part of the operator, permanent results can always be obtained, and without scarring. The same operator is equipped to remove moles. Unsightly moles should usually be removed, not only for cosmetic but for health reasons. Sometimes a mole will show signs of rapid growth; this condition should always be reported to your doctor.

YOUR MAKE-UP

As far back as 500 B.C., wise old Confucius said, "Everything has beauty, but not everyone *sees* it." This is precisely why I urge women to use modern make-up skillfully, creatively, to enhance good points and tone down bad points. Make-up, so used, can take at least ten years from any face; it can boost the morale and give the mature woman the assurance of ageless comeliness. Do not strive for glamour. Instead, strive for symmetry and harmony, for glow rather than glare. The secret of success in make-up is to *underdo* it, so that a natural effect results. Radiance, rather than pink-and-white prettiness, is your aim. Here is the finest guide to mature beauty that I can give you: *whatever happens, do not let the light go out in your face.*

With added years, the skin tends to lose the oiliness of youth; oily creams and powder foundations must be used more liberally and consistently to offset this loss. Determine which of the three basic skin colorings is yours, and have all your cosmetics keyed to your natural coloring. The coloring of the chest and shoulder area will most accurately guide you, as exposure to sun and weather change the coloring of the face. The average American woman's coloring is of the "brownette" type, a neutral beige tone.

Select a foundation cream (it *must* be of the creamy lotion type) which is the color of your skin or a shade darker. Apply it lightly and evenly over the face, throat, neck, and around the ears, using the tips of your fingers to blend it into the skin. Properly applied, it does the same thing a soft veil does: it creates a gentleness, removes harshness, youthifies instantly. Also, it protects and moistens the skin all day long. Wipe off excessive spots with your fingers, always—never with tissues which cause streaking and spoil the blended, natural look.

Now the background is on. "Let there be light." Bring out the lustre of your eyes, beginning with

YOUR EYEBROWS

Use a small toothbrush night and morning to shape the brows. Brush them "the wrong way," then straight up; then merely draw the brush along the top edge. Use a bit of ointment to keep them pliable. If the brow line is out of balance and uneven, you may need to tweeze the unruly hairs for a well-groomed outline. Remember that the most beautiful eyes are spaced so that in the distance between them another eye could be set. Widen the space between your eyebrows, if necessary; it will make you look more youthful, happy and serene.

In general your brows should be shaped like the wing of a bird, the thickest part toward the center, arching up and out. Extend your browline at the outer end, if necessary, to keep the line UP (all downward lines are aging). If your brows need accent, use a well-sharpened brow pencil and make short, hairline, *upward* strokes to form a natural-looking arch. If your brows need color, make the emphasis a little stronger on the arch. Now use the brush again (clean it with tissue after each using) in light upward strokes, to blend and diffuse, as Nature does.

YOUR EYELASHES

The fringe of protection Nature furnishes the eye does fade, and the softest, most natural addition of accent is achieved, not with mascara (which the mature woman should use sparingly, if at all) but with an eyebrow crayon applied in the so-called Garbo technique:

Apply a bit of eye crème to the upper lid *immediately* above the roots of the lashes. Now draw a line with your crayon (black for the brunette and brownette; dark brown for the blond) working the crayon well in between the lashes with short up-down strokes. This will need practice but it is worth it. Now, with a clean finger, in the same motion clean the eyelid, leaving the penciling to adhere only to the roots of the lashes, which now look twice as thick, longer, and make your eyes seem larger, more opened and alert. Now, if you wish, apply your eyelash curler, for another upward, youthful line. This famous Garbo technique is simple after you have done it a few times. Properly done, it is unnoticeable; your friends observe only that your eyes have a more pleasing expression of warmth and sincerity.

EYE SHADOW

More than any feature, the eyes tend to retain their pristine color; it is decreased vitality, lack of zest for life, that sometimes leads to the impression that they have faded. The mature woman should investigate the really beautiful interest-restoring effects of a bit of eye shadow, chosen to complement the iris, blended well with the finger to warm the oils, and then applied sparingly with the finger to the outer half of the upper eyelid. This minimizes the darker area of the lower eyelid and intensifies the color of the iris, resulting in more radiant eyes. Learn to do as much for your eyes as you do for the rest of your face. Remember that "eyes are the barometer of age."

YOUR MOUTH

A generous mouth is an index of youth and vitality; with proper make-up, you can do wonders. Your lip line will take its pattern from your brow line. These two lines, with that of the coiffure line, must be in harmony, and much has been done in recent years in cleverly reshaping mouths with a brush.

If you do not have a lipstick brush, get one tomorrow—a good sable one. Fill the brush well with lipstick, as an artist fills his brush with oils. Start from the outer corner and work toward the center; with practice, you can accomplish the line in one sweep. Then the other side; then the lower lip. When you have made the frame, you can fill it in easily. Most mature women need to extend the upper lip line in a rounder, fuller curve, and if you go over your own lip line, it is wise to powder over your mouth first to make sure any moisture is absorbed. In any case, the first requisite in preventing lipstick from spreading and fading is to have the lips perfectly dry to begin with. Aim for an amiable mouth—a happy mouth—one which gives your face an expression of hope and anticipation.

ROUGE

If you need rouge, by all means use a bit of soft cream rouge in a delicate rosy shade, well blended between the finger tips to release the oils. Smile, and then place the tiny dot of blended rouge in the center of the "smile mound." Then, with a clean finger, blend up and out; and please *underdo* it. Better no rouge at all than an unnatural, painted-looking, sharp splotch of color. Never use the old-fashioned dry cake rouge and never apply rouge with a puff, but with the fingers, "skin on skin." Use just a suspicion to start with; you can always add more. And do not make the mistake of adding a little extra rouge when you feel tired; it will make you look older, not younger. This is the general rule: never rouge lower than the ear lobe (*do* delicately rouge the ear lobes, if you wish), and never closer to the nose than in a line with the pupil of the eye as you look straight ahead.

POWDER

Select one of the wonderful new nondrying face powders in your skin-tone color (or a shade darker, for daytime wear) but with a rosy tinge, not yellowish. Be careful, too, of powders that turn yellow on the skin. Of the many rose-rachel tones available, it will repay you to be meticulously careful in selecting the one that is exactly right for you. Do not be rushed into buying the wrong shade of powder. Also, do not buy powder under artificial light; it is impossible to select the correct shade.

The manner of applying powder can make or mar. Remember that powder *sets* your make-up, so be sure that all is perfectly blended before applying it. Then shake the powder in your box to loosen it, use a fresh square of cotton about five inches square and fairly thick, dip it into the loose powder and try not to wad it down. Then, making the skin surface taut by doing facial gymnastics (much as a man does when he is shaving), roll the powder firmly and generously on, beginning with the neck.

Take your time. Powder over your eyebrows and right up to the hairline, pressing, never rubbing the powder into the skin. Continue the facial gymnastics; you can make the under-eye area taut by looking up; do not neglect it and the sides of the bridge of your nose where shadows lurk. Let the powder set for a few minutes and you are ready for the most important part of all: brush and burnish off the excess powder with the reverse side of the puff. While you do this, make the skin taut just as you did in putting on the powder. At least half the effectiveness and naturalness of your make-up will depend on doing your facial gymnastics while you put your powder *on and off*. This is because the fine lines in the skin are made shallow when the skin is made taut, and its surface is made smoother. This gentle dusting-off process should take at least two minutes. Finish by stroking the fine downy hair on the cheeks *down*.

Finally, use your eyebrow brush again to remove any excess of powder in brows and lashes. If you have long eyelashes, touch their tips with a good mascara (mascara only accentuates shortness). You may have removed a bit of brow line while removing excess powder, so lightly repair the brows and retrace the lip line if you like more color. Your make-up is finished. Was it not worth ten minutes? It should not take longer, and will need very little attention the rest of the day or evening.

YOUR PERFUME

On the subject of perfumes, which have become so much a part of the daily make-up, I am happy to note that natural flower fragrances are again coming into their own. These dainty, feminine scents are suited to any age and are an especial boon to the mature woman. From the wide range of light flowery or spicy perfumes available, you may wish to use only one and make it an expression of your own personality; or you may like the notion of using different scents for your different moods. Either way, it is a matter of personal preference, and either can be in delightful good taste. Whatever your taste in perfume, it should always be applied directly to the skin (not to the clothing)—the ear lobes, behind the ears, wrists, or, for lasting effect, on the chest area. Apply perfume lightly, lest it become overpowering. If you use perfume, buy a good one; nothing can be so destructive of personality as cheap scents. Buy it in small quantity and keep it tightly stoppered when not in use, to prevent evaporation. If you cannot include expensive perfumes in your budget, use a good toilet water or cologne. These may be used more lavishly over the body, to give a delicate lingering fragrance and garden-fresh feeling.

GOOD FEET FOR LIFE

Next to the eyes, the feet are the most abused part of the body. Many people treat their feet as if they hated them. They drive them, pinch them, punish them, shut them up in the dark, ignore them; and then wonder why their feet do not just keep on going and like it. If you have good, straight-boned, well-arched feet that cause no trouble, it is probably none of your doing. Feet are marvels of construction and resistance to neglect. If from now on you are only ordinarily decent to yours, they will respond eagerly. So will your complexion. Aching feet make wrinkles. If you doubt this, stand in front of your mirror, pretend once again that you are trying out for a part in a play, and read the line, "My feet are simply killing me."

Remember, first, that feet are bones and that the essential nutrients for good bones are plenty of calcium (milk and cheese), phosphorus (more milk), vitamin C (citrus fruits), and vitamin D (sunshine). Remember that last item particularly. So few older people give their feet an opportunity to see daylight, let alone sunlight. Go barefoot whenever you can. Give your feet sun and air and freedom from the constriction of shoes. Get them higher than your head in the Body Slant position, for at least fifteen minutes a day; they will tingle afterward and probably think it is your birthday.

If you have problem feet, take them to a good podiatrist who can give you amazing relief. Never use an arch support unless it is prescribed by an expert. Have calluses, corns, bunions, ingrown toenails corrected by a chiropodist. Spend money on your feet; it will pay better dividends in youthfulness than a facial massage, a fancy necktie, or an afternoon at the races.

My own favorite remedy for troublesome feet is a rather unusual combination—dancing and water. Good dancers must have good feet; nothing so strengthens flat and tired feet as walking on the toes. Try this to music in your room, or, still better, on the beach. Walk on your toes for 5 minutes. Then let warm water run over your feet for 2 minutes, followed by cold water for 1 minute. Do this the next time your "feet are simply killing you," and you will thank me.

Resolve, from now on, to treat your feet like the faithful friends they are. Do not undermine them with run-down heels, betray them with heelless and toeless shoes that give them no support, double-cross them with bargain shoes that do not quite fit, or torture them with high heels that tilt them too far forward. Evidence is piling up that bad footgear can be the cause of serious ligamentous and bone injury which can cause rheumatism and arthritis. Wear sturdy, well-constructed shoes with low or medium heels in the daytime; wear corrective shoes cheerfully if you need them; they are not ugly nowadays. Remember that it is not your shoes but how you walk—briskly, erectly, confidently— that indicates your youthfulness. And I want you to walk and walk and walk—with long, long steps—everywhere, every day of your long life.

THE BATH

"Water contains great healing power," said Father Kneipp, and today in Woerishofen, Bavaria, this inspired priest's "water cure" attracts thousands of people from all over the world. There you may see a group of men and women wading knee-deep in the cool fresh streams. According to Father Kneipp's theory, the fresh "alive" water brings better circulation to the feet and legs and the organs of the abdominal region. You may also see another group holding their arms, up to the shoulders, in cool running water in pine wood troughs, to create better circulation for the upper part of the body, especially the heart and lungs.

You will find the scientific counterpart of Father Kneipp's "water cure" in many of our modern hospitals where hydrotherapy (water therapy), given in tubs, tanks, pools, and specially designed showers, is a standard procedure in overcoming the effects of many diseases and disabling accidents.

Whether or not we agree that water has healing power, we do know that it is a marvelous medium for pepping up lazy circulation when applied to the feet, face, or entire body. And we know that better circulation means a better blood supply, a better blood stream rich in all the bodily nutrients, bringing good wherever it flows.

It is for this reason that I would like to establish a new "Order of the Bath," a new interest in the efficacy of water. Not just the Saturday night soak or the daily shower, but many other baths which can be of great value in our Look Younger, Live Longer program. No people are so ideally equipped for modern bathing as we Americans with our modern bathrooms. With a little ingenuity and practice you can use your bathroom for all sorts of refreshing and youthifying baths. There are two schools of the bath; tub devotees and shower addicts. Since it is easier to relax in the tub, I shall emphasize tub baths.

THE ALTERNATING BATH

My favorite bath, which thousands of my students also have enjoyed, is the Wechsel-Bad or alternating bath. I recommend this highly, especially to those whose circulation needs stimulating or those who take one cold after another.

Simply lie and relax to your heart's content in a tub of pleasantly warm water. Put a small rubber pillow under your head, if you like. Do your relaxing exercises or the Stomach Lift. (There is definite additional benefit from exercises done under warm water.) If your skin is dry, make doubly sure that the water is not too hot. Add a teaspoon of fine bath oil. You can soap and scrub while you are soaking. Use a good super-fatted toilet soap. Yogurt soap is rich and creamy, and makes you feel like Anna Held in one of her famous milk baths.

After you are clean and relaxed (and this is important) let half the warm water run out. As the warm water runs away, turn on the cold water full force. Then lie back, and with both hands mix the cold water with the remaining warm water. Keep mixing, while the water gets cooler and cooler and cooler. In three minutes your whole body will tingle and glow. You will feel refreshed and *not at all cold*. Have one of those immense bath towels ready and wrap yourself in it. Rub yourself dry, or, if you have the time, wrap the towel around you, go to bed and cover up; and relax, relax, let go of all your real or imaginary burdens.

THE SITZ BATH

This can be of immense benefit as a "pepper-upper" and requires only about five minutes. At the water resorts of Carlsbad it is called the sitz bath. At Father Kneipp's resort in Bavaria it is known as the "youth bath," perhaps because the increased circulation it gives helps to keep one young.

Fill your bathtub half way with cool (not cold) water and sit into it *sideways* of the tub, with your legs and feet hanging over the side. Does this sound silly? I assure you that it is not. The purpose of this bath, and the secret of its benefit, is that it gives specific stimulation to the important glands and organs of elimination in the lower part of the body. So important is this bath to counteract fatigue, to overcome lazy elimination, to stop an oncoming headache, and to our Look Younger, Live Longer program generally, that I cannot recommend it too highly. I look forward to the day when American bathrooms will have small sitz-bath tubs in addition to the regulation tub.

Take this bath once or twice a week or whenever you feel the need for a lift. Let the sitz bath take the place of pink pills, pale pills, benzedrine, and other harmful stimulants. After you have enjoyed the cool sitz bath awhile, you can gradually lower the temperature of the water. Soon you will enjoy it in cold water straight from the tap.

THE HERBAL BATH

This is especially good for older people. Into pleasantly warm water, put a bundle of your favorite herbs from the garden, or a tablespoonful of pine, eucalyptus, or mint, which are especially relaxing. Be sure that the water is not too hot, and you will find a fifteen-minute herbal soak exceptionally soothing to irritated nerves.

THE OIL BATH

We need soap and water for bathing, to remove dust and grime from our bodies; unfortunately, we also remove the natural body oils with it. Dry skin is becoming too prevalent, in our bath-conscious modern world. Women have learned to cream and oil their faces after washing, and their hands, but only a few are wise enough to oil their bodies after the bath.

If you have dry skin, by all means add a tablespoon of thin olive oil to your bath water. If the budget permits, get one of the exquisite bath oils that leave a fine film of oil all over the body and help to give you a younger and smoother skin.

THE SUN BATH

In Switzerland today, sun-bathing is done seriously and scientifically, due to the influence of Dr. Auguste Rollier, a prominent surgeon who fell in love with a nurse suffering tuberculosis. Determined to cure her, he left his hospital in Bern and took her high up in the Swiss Alps where the sun is at its best. There with the help of sun baths he slowly but surely accomplished her cure. Today, up in Leysin in the Swiss Alps, thousands of people come from all over the world to find health, and this same Dr. Rollier is still accomplishing amazing things.

The Rollier technique of sun-bathing is especially adapted to our Look Younger, Live Longer, program because it is gentle and easy to apply. Dr. Rollier absolutely forbids older people to take uncontrolled sun baths. When overdone, some of the rays of the sun can be positively dangerous. First of all, that part of the body which is to be exposed to the sun is oiled with a cream that filters out most of the harmful rays. Second, the head is *never* exposed but always covered or shaded. And the duration of the sun bath for older or sickly people is never more than fifteen minutes.

Here is the most important part of the Rollier sun bath technique: only the legs are exposed for the first few days. The upper part of the body is covered with a towel or a shirt. When the legs have a glowing color, then and then only is the upper part of the body exposed. There again, the abdomen and chest are exposed only for fifteen minutes for the first two days. The same procedure is applied to the back and the buttocks.

When the whole body, back and front, is fairly pink and glowing, sun baths can be extended to thirty minutes for three or four days. After that, you can work it up to one hour, but not more; Dr. Rollier has found excessive sun-bathing weakening. At all times, the head should be covered to prevent the possibility of sunstroke.

The best time to take sun baths is around ten o'clock in the morning. The least desirable time is at noon. If you can, go to the seashore and get the combined benefits of sun and water. If you cannot, do manage to let the sun caress your body, not through a window pane, but directly. The sun, like water, has magnificent healing and youthifying power and it is free for the taking. If you cannot go to the beach, why not arrange a small place on your porch or in your bedroom and on sunny days take these short, stimulating and invigorating Rollier sun baths? Start now, and you too will become an enthusiastic "sun worshipper." The sun is one of the most potent forces for our Look Younger, Live Longer program.

THE AIR BATH

"Just as fish need water, so man needs air," said Dr. Benedict Lust, a medical doctor who also practiced and applied the natural sciences at his Florida sanatorium. In big cities where people live closely together and apartments are small, there is little opportunity to give the body the chance to breathe freely of good fresh air. Yet even busy city people can take air baths at night in the privacy of their bedroom. Fortunately, pajamas and nightgowns are becoming thinner, briefer, and more porous. But why not go all the way, and sleep "in the raw"? Try it, the next time you go to bed feeling dead-tired. You will be amazed at how much fresher you feel the next morning.

In our Look Younger, Live Longer program, let us try to keep our bodies surrounded with fresh, crisp air. Take air baths, in the raw, or in the airiest of sleeping garments. Sleep in well-ventilated bedrooms. Wear light, porous clothing. And live outdoors whenever possible.

SEA BATHING

Everyone knows that this is wonderful, that it prolongs youthfulness and life. If you live near the ocean, be glad of it and make use of it. Are you afraid of the water? Learn to swim. One of my People, the beloved Annie Laurie, a brilliant San Francisco newspaperwoman, learned to swim at seventy. "What are you afraid of?" a Honolulu fisherman challenged her. "The sea, she is your mother; lie on her and she will caress and carry you." And I am delighted that bathing suits are getting briefer. The briefer the better, for our sun- and air-starved bodies.

THE DRY BATH

In France, where it is very popular, this is called the friction bath. Its value lies in the fact that it is soothing and quieting. You can obtain a coarse bath glove made of twisted wool and horsehair in any of the better drugstores, and it will prove a good investment for one whose nerves need quieting or who wishes to have baby-smooth skin all over.

With the glove on the right hand, proceed gently to rub the feet, calves, thighs and abdomen with a circular motion. Then change the glove to the left hand and gently massage the rest of the body. You will be surprised to find how soothing and relaxing this bath can be. In France it is taken before retiring and is proclaimed an excellent remedy for sleeplessness. In hot weather, French people sprinkle a pleasant eau de cologne on the glove which is not only a mild deodorizer but also helps to remove dead, dry skin from the body.

For the rest of your long life, let your bath be not merely a daily habit but a daily ritual. Join the new "Order of the Bath" and get as much as possible out of it, for health's sake as well as for beauty and cleanliness. Instead of rushing through a "necessary" procedure, take time for the particular type of bath that suits your need or mood, and give yourself the full benefit of it.

This is a good time for women to brush their hair well, tie it back and give their faces a chance to soak up cleansing cream. Bath time is the time for applying deodorants, for shaving or applying depilatories to the underarms and legs. These matters should be attended to more, rather than less, scrupulously as women grow older. And this is the time for attention to toenails and fingernails; your pedicure is as important as your manicure.

If you do not have a full-length mirror in your bathroom, order one tomorrow. Make friends with your entire body for the rest of your long life. A body sags, at any age, when it is discouraged. Who has been discouraging your body? You have. By looking at it only to see what is wrong, what is changing, what is lost. By looking at it only to cover up its defects as quickly as possible with clothing. By not looking at it at all, perhaps. That is the unkindest cut.

After your bath, do not hurry into your clothing. Look at yourself in the mirror. Let your body know that you value it. Talk to yourself. Remind yourself of what you have learned: that plenty of yellow and green vegetables and other vitamin A foods will make your skin alive and radiant from the inside; plenty of milk, yogurt, raw vegetables, and sunshine (calcium, phosphorus and vitamin D) will nourish your bones and keep your body straight and youthfully erect; and plenty of proteins (lean meat, eggs and cheese) will improve your muscle tone.

Do not take your bath at the same time every day. Doing the same thing at the same time too regularly is "elderly." Plan your bath for a time when you have nothing else to do for at least an hour. Follow it, if possible, with fifteen minutes in the Body Slant position. I cannot suggest too often that you invest in a good strong board that does not sag in the middle and is comfortable enough so that you will be able to relax or do the Stomach Lift. Relax, relax. Let your own blood flow. Do the Stomach Lift. One, pull in. Two, pull in more. Three, pull in and flatten still more. Keep the muscles tense for about ten counts, then let go, relax. Do this ten times and know that you are permanently flattening your abdomen, taking inches off your waist, and giving your whole body firmness, youthfulness and dignity.

CLOTHES

Now I am going to lay down the law. After fifty, no bright red. For women, no bright-red hats, dresses, shoes. For men, no bright-red neckties either in solid colors or splashy designs. Why? Because bright red is an emotion. It screams aloud. After fifty, it screams one of three things:

"Look at me; I am old but I don't admit it."

"Look at me; I am old but I can distract your attention from the fact."

"Look at me; I am old but I am really very young at heart."

In short, the person who wears bright red after fifty is saying to the world, "Look at me; I am old."

In the Look Younger, Live Longer program, we are not old. Moreover, we are secure in our agelessness. We wear plenty of bright red, but we wear it inside us, pumping from our hearts, coursing through our arteries, radiating out to our muscles and to the surfaces of our skin from head to foot. The world knows by looking at us that we are youthful. We have nothing to deny, nothing to distract attention from, nothing to prove.

To a lesser degree, be wary of taking refuge in wearing gray, which says, "I am old and I admit it." Use navy blue, black and white. The smartest women in the world, regardless of age, concentrate on these colors. Use accents of crisp, spotless white with your navy and black. In summer, try wearing all white. Spotless gloves, whether of cotton or the finest kid, are an indispensable accessory.

The well-dressed woman is never "fancy." Neither is she extravagant; her clothes can be few and inexpensive. Mrs. Harrison Williams, the fabulous "Mona," who for years has headed the list of best-dressed women, surprised us all by announcing that her budget for clothes was a comparatively modest one. Line and cut are more important than the material from which the dress is made.

Two of my best-dressed friends, the Duchess of Windsor and Lady Mendl, wear clothes of very simple design (both are clients of Mainbocher). Lady Mendl's "little girl" dress is almost a uniform with her. The upper part is loose-fitting with a round neck and three-quarter length sleeves, the full skirt is drawn in at the waist with a cord or a small belt, and there are two little pockets concealed in the folds of the skirt. (And *always*, she wears white gloves.) The Duchess of Windsor wears clothes of similar simplicity and accents them with her beautiful jewels. The last time I saw her we discussed clothes and she agreed with me that the best-dressed women do not follow "the fashion" but rather stick to the lines and colors that are most becoming to them and make but few concessions to the "style" of the moment. Smart women everywhere adapt their clothes to themselves and never blindly follow any "new" or "old" look.

Your personality is your most precious possession. What you wear, and how you wear it, can be a beautiful expression of your own personality or an unbeautiful imitation of another's. You can be a creative artist in terms of your own personality, and translate the ideal image of yourself into reality. But remember that eccentricity is not chic, and it is not chic to be "too chic."

Make a point of knowing your own figure; the woman with a "perfect" figure is rare indeed. The length of the neck, size of the head, set of the shoulders, size and position of the bust, breadth of shoulders and hips, length of waist and of arms and legs, must be given proportionate consideration in relation to each other.

Be critical about the cut of a garment. Far better one garment of burlap properly cut and fitted, than twenty dresses of the richest fabric poorly designed and put together. Remember that it is not quantity of clothes that makes the well-dressed woman; you can buy dresses by the dozen and still be one of the world's worst-dressed women.

If you can afford to have clothes especially designed for you, then you have no excuse for being dowdy, or overdressed. If you plead "can't afford it," I say you have even less excuse, for then you surely cannot afford to waste money on clothing that does not do well by you. Learn something about dress designing and making. Learn about yourself; you can be economically well dressed for the rest of your life.

Learn about color and what it can do *to* you or *for* you. What color are your eyes? Your hair? Your skin? These are your guides. Does the color of your clothing distort your self-coloring, or subtly flatter it? Is your present wardrobe a hit-or-miss collection of clashing colors? Snatched-up "bargains" that make no bargain of you? Learn to plan ahead of your purchases. Start with one basically good garment in your best basic color and line. Add harmonious companion pieces as you are able to. Restrict bright colors to accessories that add a small lilting note to the suave harmony of *you*. Beautiful scarves, handkerchiefs, costume jewelry, flowers, discreetly applied can be inexpensive grace notes expressing the "inner woman."

Avoid, as you would the plague, anything gaudy. Nothing so quickly stamps the ill-dressed woman as a profusion of attire which screams for attention. On New York's fashionable Fifth Avenue you can see swarms of such misguided females, any day of the week. Clad in a riotous profusion of stuffs, teetering on gaudy slippers, clattering an astonishing load of costume baubles; "over-Saksed" as the punsters put it, to the total loss of their own personalities.

If you are going to live a long life of agelessness, plan an ageless wardrobe. Unsuitable and unbecoming clothing can age your whole appearance. Wisely selected, it can take years off your looks. Strive for *under*statement. Simplicity of line and cut know no age and never go out of style.

I insist that there is no such thing as a "stylish stout." Stoutness is forever unhealthy, unstylish and unnecessary. If you have allowed yourself to become overweight, get your waistline down again. Flatten it. Strengthen it. Make it your aim in life to keep your muscles so strong and elastic that you can free yourself permanently from that one-piece harness called the corset. Your own, natural "muscular corset" is the best of all undergarments. Grandma Reynolds achieved it in her eighties, and you can too.

Give time and thought to discovering your own best style and be true to it for the rest of your long life. It will be suitable to the needs of your way of life; pleasant to look upon; comfortable to wear; and a true expression of your self. It can make you, no matter where or who you are, a well-dressed woman of the world.

As for men, darker suits are the general rule and the most practical for working hours in the city. No need to be sombre about it though; there are shades of blue, gray, and brown that are dark enough for wear in a sooty city without having funereal aspects. If you cannot indulge in a large wardrobe, concentrate on navy blue and gray; they are your best colors. Do not be afraid to wear a snappy blue flannel suit with a bold white chalk stripe; you will look younger and feel younger in such a suit.

And gray flannel slacks with a well-cut tweed jacket can be worn almost any place during the daytime. Insist on a youthful cut; and why not give up vests? Avoid "off colors" in tans, light blues, greens or mixtures. I call these gallstone colors because they make one look as if he had jaundice.

You may economize on the number of suits you have, but never at the expense of their tailoring. Two expertly tailored suits will give far more satisfaction in long wear and good appearance than will four poorly tailored ones.

Neckties can make or break your claim to being a well-dressed man. I believe hand-painted ties are my pet aversion. They scream, "I am rich, but I do not know what to do with my money." Let discretion be your guide. Plain ties in neutral colors are always good taste. Small dots, narrow stripes, or small allover patterns in subdued colors take second place. Beware of gaudy, parrot-like colors and screaming patterns; they scream of immaturity. Best of all, wear a maroon, gray, or blue tie with your navy blue suit. Maroon, navy blue, or black ties with your gray flannels. Socks should match your tie and be in solid color. If you wear silk hose, avoid stripes or patterns. If you wear lisle or wool, a small pattern is permissible. *Always* wear a crisp white handkerchief in your breast pocket and let two or three inches of it show. A pair of brown suede shoes would be a youthful and practical addition to your wardrobe.

White shirts are unquestionably the choice of the best-dressed men; but scrupulously white. However, the growing tendency of American men toward colored shirtings in subdued shades can be a pleasant and practical note, when used with discretion. While frowned upon for after-dark wear in town, this tendency has achieved some standing for daytime attire. Shirt collars are very important. The height and cut of a collar can add to, or subtract from, your age. A higher cut for a thin neck, and a low cut for a plump or normal neck.

Naturally, your problems are few if you have retained a youthful body. If you have permitted yourself to grow fat or have developed a "bay window," start to get rid of it at once. (If Grandma Reynolds did it, you certainly can.) Make the *Bauchgymnastik* a daily habit. In the meantime, you can help matters considerably by wearing one of the elastic "supporters" which can be purchased in any drugstore.

Men's clothes, while much more comfortable than they were a few years ago, are still badly in need of reform. The starched white collar, the pointed-toe shoe, and the derby hat are becoming almost nonexistent. In their place we have the more comfortable, collar-attached soft shirts, more comfortable shoes, the comparatively new moccasin, and no hats at all. Our great need, however, is for a glorified coverall, a one-piece garment to take the place of the present coat and trousers. I believe the time is not far off when men will wear clothes resembling those developed by the air force during the war. They are extremely comfortable, practical and attractive. I am glad to see that in summer and in year-round warm climates, men of all ages are being emancipated from slavery to their dark suits. Slack suits in light-weight materials and lighter colors are most appropriate for our increasing leisure hours.

For men and women both, I would lay down one final law: whatever you wear, let it be *always* well-pressed, well-brushed, and scrupulously clean.

SECTION THREE

YOUR GOOD LIFE

XI. THE CONTROLLED LIFE

J HAVE SAID that in the course of my life I have met many People, that People are my great interest and that many of them are my good friends.

In my lifelong studies, I have discovered that People, whatever their talents, achievements, or position in life, have one thing in common: they make it their habit always to be at their best—to feel their best, look their best, and use their best efforts to make the world better, saner or happier. In other words, I find that People make it their habit to control themselves and their lives instead of allowing themselves to be controlled and pushed around by circumstances.

All my People are in the second half of their lives. It cannot be otherwise. A young person cannot be a Person; he can simply move in that direction, give evidence that one day he will be a Person. Young people can eat intelligently, establish good habits of hygiene, grooming and dress, establish sound patterns of living, thinking and behavior. If they do these things, well and good. But they do not know *why* they are doing them; they do not enjoy their self-control. That comes later.

Be glad that you are in the second half of life. As George Bernard Shaw, ageless at ninety-three, has said, "Youth is altogether wasted on young people." True self-control comes only with maturity. So does true self-awareness. The young person must conform, be like everyone else, to be happy. The mature person can say to himself, "I am unique. There is no one in the world who is exactly like me," and enjoy this, capitalize on it. He can say, "I love and am loved," and know what he is talking about. It is only in maturity that we have loved enough to understand and evaluate love. The mature person can say, "I am important to myself, to my family, to my community," and know wherein he is important. He can also know wherein he is unimportant; there is the great test of maturity.

Only the mature person, also, can have true self-confidence. In the first half of life, we are finding ourselves, reproducing ourselves, earning a living for ourselves and our dependents. In the second half of life, we can confidently appraise ourselves, find out who we are, what we are good for, and what we were put into the world to accomplish. We have enough confidence in our strength to be able to admit and remedy our weaknesses; enough confidence in our education to want to go on learning; enough confidence in our lives to want to go on developing, expanding, *living*.

What are the attributes of youth? They are both plus and minus. The plus attributes are: courage, curiosity, excitement. The minus attributes are: ignorance, egocentricity, overconfidence.

What are the attributes of age? Again, they are both plus and minus. The plus ones: caution, objectivity, wisdom. The minus ones: timidity, intolerance, fear of change.

Check over these attributes, both plus and minus. What do you find? You find that in some respects you are still young; that in some respects you have always been old. *You have been both young and old all of your life.* Now discard all your minuses, both of youth and of age. Make a list of all the plus attributes. Resolve, consciously and deliberately, to rule out all of the minus side and to develop all of the plus side (of both youth and age) for the rest of your long life. This is true maturity.

The French philosopher, Henri Bergson, has said, "To exist is to change, to change is to mature, to mature is to go on creating oneself endlessly."

HOW DOES ONE GAIN MATURITY?

Just as some people are lucky enough to inherit good teeth, strong bodies, and superior digestive systems, some people also have the good fortune to be born of happy, well-adjusted parents and to inherit thereby the ingredients for true maturity.

Many others achieve maturity by instinct, often by finding, either in real life or on library shelves, some great friend, teacher, guide or philosopher with whom they identify themselves, whose life they use as a model for their own lives.

Many others, unfortunately, are neither "born" to maturity, nor do they acquire it. They arrive at the second half of life still woefully immature, still fighting the old battles of their childhood against grownups who ruled or thwarted them; still tense with the insecurity and guilt of their teens; still driven by the mbitions and anxieties of their thirties. These are the "seekers," ho run from one thing to another. They are looking for help ut have not the maturity nor the wisdom to know what they ctually need. Countless such "seekers" have come to my classes and I believe that by teaching them to strengthen their bodies, especially their nerves, I have been able to help many of them.

However, many of these people need psychiatric help or psychological counseling in order to attain true maturity. I look forward to the day when regular checkups with the family psychiatrist will be as much a matter of course as checkups with the family doctor, dentist, and oculist. Modern life grows more and more complex. There is increasing need for true maturity if, in the course of our long lives, we are to meet serenely the changes, challenges and anxieties of the atomic era. We need equilibrium and assurance. I agree with that great modern philosopher, Joshua Loth Liebman, that "modern psychology can help normal people to maintain their equilibrium or to regain it." I also agree with Dr. Liebman when he adds that "religion can give both assurance and a spiritual purpose in life."

The famous psychoanalyst, Dr. Carl Jung, in Zurich, Switzerland, once said to me, "In all the thousands who come to me for help, those who have some faith, some religion, get well more quickly."

Truly mature people, wherever you find them, are spiritual people. They may or may not live according to a specific creed or faith; the important thing is that they *have* faith—faith in themselves, in their fellow-men, in the existence of a power, a universal order and purpose which is greater than themselves. This can only be achieved in the second half of life. Dr. Edward Bortz, a former president of the American Medical Association, tells us that man reaches physical maturity at 25; emotional maturity at 35; intellectual maturity at 45; but that spiritual maturity comes in the later years.

If you are falling short of true maturity, finding yourself hampered by impulses, anxieties, depressions which cannot understand or overcome, even after you have built up your physical health and strength, then by all means consult a psychiatrist or psychologist. Dr. George Lawton, a consulting psychologist specializing in the problems of later life, tells us that the aim of such counseling is "to release the individual's potentialities for growth, make him more effective in the use of his energies."

WHOM DO YOU ADMIRE?

Whether or not you need special help, follow the example of those people of whom I have spoken who have achieved maturity by identification with some mature person whom they admire. Go to your library. Read newspapers, magazines, biographies and autobiographies. Learn to know People, in present-day life and in the pages of history. Find someone whose life story kindles your imagination, someone who resembles yourself in interests, in point of view, in his or her way of attacking a job. Identify yourself with this Person.

I do *not* mean that you should imitate this Person, become a carbon copy, a poseur. Pose is hideous. Identifying oneself with a specific individual, on the other hand, can be constructive. It impresses your subconscious mind with a tendency in the direction of achievement and strength.

Identify yourself with a Person who perhaps shares your handicap. Everyone has a handicap, either real or imaginary. Some are too tall, some too short, some suffer from poor physique, poor vision, poor hearing, shyness, speech defects, poor muscular co-ordination. Some have big noses, big hands, big feet. Some are handicapped by money and social position, and some by being born on the wrong side of the tracks. Some think themselves too ugly, and some think themselves too good-looking. I have met not a few men who suffered acutely from having been called, "Hey, handsome!" all their lives.

Now say to yourself, "I—this person sitting here in this chair —I am a Person. I could do what this similar Person whom I admire has done—

If I had his talents
If I had his training
If I had his opportunities."

Psychologists agree that the majority of people reach middle life without having begun to explore their potentialities. You have talents and capacities for development, of which so far you have only dreamed. Training is yours for the asking, whether you wish to go to college, as my friend Grandma Reynolds did at 60; or like another 60-year-old student of mine, take a free course in ceramics in the Adult Education Department of your nearest public school. You may not be "discovered" by Hollywood, as Grandma Reynolds was, but you will certainly be discovered by your community. You may not make a small fortune in decorative pottery, as my other student has done, but on the other hand, you may!

"You can look the way you want to look, if you want to steadily enough," as my friend Mrs. Astaire has demonstrated. Also, you can be the Person you want to be, if you want to steadily enough. Whatever your age, you can be what you want to be. Opportunity keeps right on knocking, day in and day out.

For a magnificent example of life lived to the full for almost a hundred years, read books by and about Dr. Lillian J. Martin of California. In her youth, Dr. Martin taught high school chemistry. In her thirties, she went to Germany to study psychology (then a new science), took a professorship at Leland Stanford University, made ten fresh contributions to psychological research and then was retired, in the natural order of things, at the age of sixty-five.

Did Dr. Martin "retire"? Assuredly not. She then *began* her great work. Believing that the secret of youthfulness lay in breaking with the old and tackling the new, she launched into child guidance work and opened the first mental hygiene clinic for pre-school children in San Francisco. Working with children, she became interested in their grandparents also. Then she opened an Old Age Clinic in San Francisco, now world-famous, with branches in Los Angeles and New York City.

Dr. Martin learned to type at 65. She learned to drive a car in her seventies. At 75 she went alone to Russia. At 81 she toured Mexico alone in her car. At 88 she made a tour of South America, including a journey up the Amazon. At 89 she managed a 64-acre farm (at a profit) with four 60-year-old helpers.

If you are interested in art or architecture, read about Anna Mary Robertson Moses of Eagle Bridge, New York; and Frank Lloyd Wright of Spring Green, Wisconsin. Grandma Moses took up painting seriously at the age of 76. She has had more than 35 exhibitions; some of her canvases have sold for $3,000. Recently, at the age of 88, she was awarded the Women's National Press Club award "for outstanding contribution to contemporary thought and achievement." Grandma Moses says (and artist friends of mine have corroborated this), "Anyone can paint who wants to. All you have to do is get the brush and paint and start in."

Frank Lloyd Wright was little known as an architect in his youth and middle life. At the age of 80, he is world-famous and recently received the highest professional honors from the American Institute of Architects. His comment on age is, "A creative life is a young one. What makes everyone think that 80 is old?"

A gold medal for distinguished service to humanity has recently been awarded to Dr. Lillian M. Gilbreth—engineer, psychologist and author—by the National Institute of Social Sciences. Dr. Gilbreth is in her seventies. She is an engineer, psychologist, and professor; also mother of twelve children, author of ten books, recipient of nine academic degrees, and an industrial consultant now presiding over her own corporation.

At 82, Mrs. Anita McCormick Blaine of Chicago, not content with years of active interest in public affairs, progressive education and world government, has just launched New York City's newest newspaper.

At 87, Connie Mack is one of baseball's outstanding managers.

At 79, Dorothy Dix still gives modern, nationally heeded advice to the lovelorn.

At 75, Winston Churchill is called "a young man with a bright future," a leader in the affairs of Europe and the world, and, in his spare time, an excellent painter.

At 90, John Dewey is America's greatest philosopher.

At 75, Albert Schweitzer, honored, revered and beloved by the entire civilized world, has made outstanding contributions to humanity as a scholar, theologian, musician, writer, lecturer, philosopher and physician, and, in his missionary hospital in French Equatorial Africa, is now devoting himself tirelessly to the direct service of mankind.

Past 80, Arturo Toscanini, symphonic orchestra conductor, is the "maestro" unsurpassed in energy and vitality.

Billie Burke, who in her twenties was called "America's favorite redhead," is still being called that, forty years later. Gay, youthful, perennial, she is now an author as well as a movie star, and declares that she still stands on her head and turns somersaults every morning before breakfast. This seems natural enough, since she is my friend and one of my favorite People, and a few years ago wrote glowingly of my diets which, she said, "have given pleasure and comfort to so many."

It was only in the second half of life that Benjamin Franklin became famous. He was past 80 when he wrote his famous *Autobiography*.

Clara Barton, founder of the American Red Cross, lived actively until the age of 91.

Sophocles wrote *Oedipus Rex* at 90.

Oliver Wendell Holmes wrote *Over the Teacups* at 85.

Titian painted his greatest masterpiece at 85, and lived to be 99.

The immortal Ninon de Lenclos has been called one of the most significant, as well as one of the most beautiful women of the seventeenth century. A contemporary of her later years wrote of her: "Until she was over 60, she had lovers who loved her greatly and the most virtuous people of France for her friends. Until she was 90 she was sought by the best society of her time."

There is no limit to the proof that, as life goes on, energy can and does *increase*. Examples are limitless of men and women who, in the second half of their lives, have found their energy heightened, their creative powers intensified, their ability to learn doubled and redoubled. Wherever we look we find examples not just of continuing productivity, but of the new flowering of gifts, talents and abilities at 40, 60, and beyond.

What is the secret? Let me repeat it:

Good health.
A strong, vibrant body.
A positive attitude of mind.

I spoke earlier of the international celebrity, Elsie de Wolfe Mendl, a good friend and faithful student of nutrition, of whom I am very proud. In the first half of her life, Elsie de Wolfe was an actress. Born in a house which stood on the present site of Macy's department store (she likes to say she was born in Macy's basement), she was educated abroad, presented at Queen Victoria's court, and moved in the inner circle of the glittering society of the Edwardian Era, in the United States and Europe. However, with the death of her father it became necessary to find some means of support for her mother and herself.

Elsie de Wolfe had always loved amateur theatricals, and she turned now to the professional stage for her living. David Belasco coached her. Charles Frohman was her producer. Later, she was star and manager of her own company. She starred with Sir Johnston Forbes-Robertson, John Drew, the Barrymores, Maude Adams, and many others. She was known as "the best-dressed woman on the American stage."

With her friend Elizabeth Marbury, with whom she shared houses in New York and in Versailles, just outside of Paris, Elsie de Wolfe became an internationally famous hostess as well. Her parties were breathtaking; her friends were kings and queens, princesses, diplomats, poets, painters, musicians, writers, admirals, generals, and stars of opera, stage and screen.

One day she walked from the stage, through the wings, into her dressing room and sat down before the mirror to remove her make-up. Suddenly she heard, clearly and distinctly, the voice of her inner self saying, "Those are the last words you will ever speak in the theatre." She had always listened to her inner voice, sometimes even talked back to it. Now she said to herself, aloud, "All right. What are you afraid of?" And began to plan another career.

From earliest childhood, Elsie de Wolfe had hated ugliness. It was associated in her mind with the drawing room of her parents' house which was indeed ugly, "done" in the height of mid-Victorian elegance—tassels, lambrequins, depressing tan wallpapers with splotchy red-and-gray designs. She had made her life a quest for beauty. In the world of society and the theatre, she had learned to create beauty for herself, learned the arts of dress and make-up, studied her own good and bad points and learned what to play up and what to play down.

Ugliness in her surroundings had always depressed her. Always conscious of rooms, she knew instinctively what was right or wrong about them. Closing her eyes in an ugly room (and in those days, the more lavish the room, the uglier it was), she would mentally re-create it and make it beautiful.

When Elsie de Wolfe decided to leave the theatre and become an interior decorator for the second half of her life, she was, therefore, turning back to a childhood dream. With no special training, no capital, nothing but many friends and an indomitable pioneering spirit, she became America's first woman interior decorator. Her first big assignment was the decoration of New York's celebrated Colony Club.

Stanford White, designer of the building, said, "Give the job of decorating to Elsie, and *let the girl alone.*" That assignment was uphill work; American women were accustomed to living in Victorian ugliness. But gradually Elsie de Wolfe won her crusade for beauty—warm, glowing colors on walls, bright chintzes in drawing rooms, indoor "garden rooms," furniture that was beautiful, useful, and comfortable, and mirrors, mirrors everywhere.

I have not space to tell you the whole story of Elsie de Wolfe, of her two careers, of her parties, friends, houses, innovations, activities, her social, personal and professional triumphs. That needs a book of its own and she herself has written it, her delightful autobiography *After All.*

Lady Mendl's husband is a distinguished Englishman, Sir Charles, for many years attached to the British Embassy in Paris.

He is an ageless gentleman with a delightful sense of humor and countless friends, usually very famous and beautiful ones. I recall as one of the most interesting occasions of my life the day in 1936 when Lady Charles Cavendish took me to one of the famous "Sunday afternoons" at Lady Mendl's villa in Versailles.

In the center of a group in which everybody was "somebody," I was received by a tiny lady, soignée, with shining dark eyes and platinum-white hair. She showed me her copy of my book, *Eat and Grow Beautiful*. It was well marked and underscored. Across the front she had written, "I *like* that man!"

Most of her life she had been interested in nutrition. As a child, she had wanted good teeth and a beautiful complexion; instinctively, she had avoided candy and other sweets. As the "best-dressed woman on the American stage," she had needed a perfect figure and had achieved it by teaching herself to like only fresh, vital foods, *under*eating always and cultivating the great art of relaxation. So important does she consider nutrition that for years her specially trained chef has traveled with her wherever she has gone. Monsieur Fraise (Mr. Strawberry—a good name for a good chef) has learned to prepare exactly the foods that Lady Mendl likes. Later on I shall give you some of his recipes.

"What is the secret of being an internationally famous hostess?" I have asked Lady Mendl. Her answer is, "Get a good chef; serve superb food." But we who know "our Elsie" know that it is her immense vitality, her love of life which has made her not only an internationally famous hostess, but one of the most adored women in the world.

Lady Mendl has long since adopted my Look Younger, Live

Longer principles. "I have originated modern styles in clothes and decoration," she tells me. "You have originated the modern manner of eating." In 1937 she gave a large party in my honor at her Paris apartment. Her guests included some of the world's most attractive women: the Duchess of Windsor, Lady Diana Manners, Lady Charles Cavendish, Mrs. Harrison Williams, Princess Karputhala. This was the first time these women had realized the limitless possibilities of good nutrition, for themselves and for the people of their countries. I gave them the first vegetable juice cocktail ever served in Paris and their enthusiasm was unbounded. The Duchess of Windsor, Lady Mendl, and my mother were the first three women in Europe to own the vegetable-juice extracting machine which was then my special innovation, and which I hope will someday be an indispensable part of household, restaurant, and hospital equipment everywhere.

Like all my People, Lady Mendl is ageless. She knows that keeping one's interests alive keeps old age from the door. Passionately devoted to France, she was active in that country's behalf during and after both World Wars. Lady Mendl is one of the few American women to have been awarded the Grand Croix de Guerre. Nowadays, in addition to maintaining her Paris apartment and villa at Versailles, she has become my neighbor in Beverly Hills, California. As always, wherever she is, her parties are wonderful; this fabulous Person is surrounded by the greatest talents, the greatest names, and the greatest minds of our time.

"The longer I live," she says, "the more I realize that it is never too late to learn. I have always been eager for the new and willing to discard the old in its favor. I never think of myself as being old. I am deeply interested in all of the new movements which are taking shape around me. I am an optimist. My favorite motto, which is embroidered on a pillow I carry with me when I travel, is 'Never complain. Never explain.'

"I have lived and laughed and loved. I have waved over my life the magic wand of self-control. I love life. I have made it an adventure. I have thrived on opposition. I rejoice that I was born with the courage to live."

XII. THE BALANCED LIFE

*Y*OU HAVE learned that the secret of good health is a balanced diet, that the secret of good looks is a balanced blood stream. What is the secret of a good life? Balanced living.

The second half of life is the time to take inventory, to balance your life just as an accountant balances his books. In fact, your own life is a book. It has a page for each day—36,500 pages. Now is the time, consciously and deliberately, to balance the book of your life.

How does it look so far? Are there blank pages in it? Do not let that dismay you. Many of the most successful lives, as we have seen, get off to a slow start. In youth, most of our decisions are made for us. Most of us must work in order to live; we take the job we can get, whether or not it is the job we wanted. We lose sight of early ambitions in the race to keep even with the monthly bills. If there are empty or unsatisfactory pages in the first half of the book of your life, now is the time to begin to balance those pages by filling the second half of your book to overflowing.

BALANCE YOUR PERSONALITY

Are you an introvert or an extrovert? An extrovert is a person whose interests are centered on external objects and actions. An introvert is a person whose interests are directed inward, who finds his satisfaction in the life of thought and fancy.

The well-balanced, mature person is neither extrovert nor introvert; he is something of both. Just as you have two sides to your body, a right and a left side, so you have two sides to your personality. You are both extrovert and introvert, active and passive, a giver and a receiver.

The circumstances of your life have decided, up till now, which side of you should be developed first. The man who has had a wife and family to support, the woman left a widow with young children, the unmarried man or woman who has assumed financial responsibility for parents or younger brothers and sisters—all have developed the "right," or active side, of their personalities. They have become doers, drivers, fighters in the competitive world.

On the other hand, women who have concerned themselves chiefly with domesticity, men and women with private incomes or with responsibility for no one except themselves, have developed the "left" side of their personalities. They have become passengers, not drivers; dreamers, not doers; spectators, not participators in the competitive struggle of life.

Whichever side of yourself has been developed by the first half of your life, well and good. Now is the time to balance your personality. This is your big opportunity, your challenge, your adventure, to release and develop the submerged side of yourself. Here is the source of new, undreamed-of stores of hidden energy, ready to be tapped. Here is the source of new ideas, new skills, new careers, new conquests, a whole new lease on life.

Has your chief concern, until now, been in getting along with other people, acquiring material possessions, dealing with facts? Learn now to get along with yourself; find an absorbing solitary hobby. Begin to think less about getting money and more about giving it away. Substitute ideas for facts.

Do you want to be alone? Find outside interests and deliberately make for yourself the opportunity to be with other people. Are your interests intellectual and spiritual, rather than material? Develop a passionate desire for a new car, a diamond bracelet, a trip to Europe—something which you cannot possibly afford—and begin methodically to earn the money for it. Do you live in an ivory tower? Find people and things in the real world that interest you—politics, the stock market, co-operative marketing, projects such as Father Flanagan's Boys Town—and delve into them, learn the facts about them.

Are you dependable, self-sufficient? Begin to let yourself depend upon others. Have you always been a "giver"? Let others have the pleasure of giving to you. Are you a talker? Begin to be a listener. A teacher? Take a course in something you know absolutely nothing about. Are you serious-minded? Seriously cultivate your frivolous side. Domestic? Take a part-time office job. Conservative? Take a deliberate risk. A creature of habit? Stay up all night occasionally, and spend the entire next day in bed. Doing the same thing at the same time is definitely "old maidish."

BALANCE YOUR MIND

The well-balanced personality is the rounded, fully developed, flexible personality. The well-balanced mind is the flexible mind. Just as you need bodily exercise to keep your body youthful, so your mind needs exercise to keep tone and muscle in your mental life. You need, as Dorothea Brande says in her book *Wake Up and Live*,* to "be able to stop one activity and turn to

---

* The rules based on those in *Wake Up and Live* by Dorothea Brande are used by permission of Simon and Schuster, publishers.

another, varying the approach and strength behind each effort with the deftness of a skillful tennis player meeting the shifting play of an opponent." Mrs. Brande suggests such exercises as these for keeping mentally agile:

Write a letter or talk for fifteen minutes a day without using the words "I, me, or mine."

Talk at length about yourself to a companion without complaining, boasting, or (if possible) without boring the companion.

Learn to think for half an hour exclusively on one subject.

Make yourself talk without such verbal mannerisms as "I mean," "As a matter of fact," "And so on."

Give yourself an occasional day in which you answer "yes" to every reasonable request.

In her valuable *Handbook for Old Age Counsellors*, Dr. Lillian J. Martin offers her own exercises for retaining mental flexibility. Here are some of them:

Plan each day; follow the plan. No two days exactly alike.

Read the newspaper each day; summarize and write down the parts that interest you.

Read aloud a few minutes daily, rapidly, to guard against a slow, "elderly" manner of speech.

Take brisk walks of exploration; when you return, write down what you recall.

Control your reveries. Listen to the radio with a pad and pencil and make a mark on the pad each time you allow your mind to wander.

To these I have added some Look Younger, Live Longer mind-limbering suggestions of my own:

Make decisions. A wrong decision is better than none at all.

Upset your opinions. Turn them inside out. Try on the other person's point of view and see how it fits.

Laugh. Laughter aids digestion and circulation and has a rejuvenating effect on the entire body as well as on the mind.

Get mad. Anger is a source of mental and emotional energy, a housecleaning. When you are good and mad, do not sit still or lie in bed; get up and walk, walk furious and fast. Do not "stew in your own juice" (it can be poisonous when you are mad).

Do not gossip. Do not chatter. Do not waste thought on unessentials.

Do not worry about your dignity. As someone has said, "It is a wise person who is willing to sound foolish."

Never stop studying. Study the books you read; mark them; take notes on them. Study the music you hear, the people you meet, the places you visit, the world you encounter.

BALANCE YOUR ACTIVITIES

The older you get, the busier you need to be. In the first half of life, you were carried along by the momentum of youth, the sheer excitement of being young. In the first half, you skimmed life's surface. In the second half, you drink deeper. You evaluate the past and estimate the future. You create your own momentum by balancing your activities and interests, by beginning, at last, to do things not just because you *must*, but because you *want* to do them.

How do you find these new interests and activities? Ask yourself the question: "What would I do if I had my life to live over again?"

Whatever you have always wanted to do, you can do *now*, in some version, some wholly satisfactory form. If you wanted to be a pianist and life made you a housewife, take piano lessons now. *Be* a pianist. Play for an audience, your family and friends, at first. But keep practising, studying, and working. See what happens. If you have always wanted to be a pianist, the chances are that you will be a competent one.

If you have no special unfulfilled dreams, turn back to your childhood, as Walter Pitkin advises in his book *The Best Years*. What did you like to do best when you were ten? Play store? Play at being an actor? Draw? Sew? Watch ants for hours on end? All right. Just for fun, get a Saturday afternoon job in the local gift shop, bookshop, or department store. Join the local Little Theatre group and collect tickets, paint scenery, etc.; eventually you will get a chance to do something better. Learn professional dressmaking or upholstery in your free evenings. Enroll in an evening school for a natural science course. Whatever you loved to do in childhood and never had a chance to do in adult life—do it now.

Build in your new activities behind your present ones. Where will you get the extra energy for this? *From doing it.* There is nothing so stimulating as balancing your activities. "Listlessness and fatigue," says Marie Beynon Ray in her book, *How Never To Be Tired*, "give way to energy and excitement when you are doing what you really want to do."

"Do the thing you fear," says Dale Carnegie, who by encouraging students of all ages to stand up and speak in public has helped many to find new self-confidence, new potentialities, new careers.

I agree with Mr. Carnegie that public speaking can be of great help as a balancer, both of personality and of activity, if one has something to say and the ability to express oneself clearly and forcefully. I urge my students, in addition to joining free-for-all discussion groups, to take writing courses to develop clear thinking and vocabulary, and voice and speech training to develop good diction, an asset which alone is worth its weight in gold. I have seen men and women transformed and revitalized, in the second half of life, by the discovery that they could organize their ideas, put them into words, and make people listen and applaud.

Balanced activity is a "must" in our Look Younger, Live Longer program. I urge my students by all means to take advantage of the modern technique of aptitude testing—scientific tests to determine such aptitudes as creative imagination, tonal memory, finger dexterity, accounting ability, structural visualization, and many others. Tests are given by Vocational Guidance Bureaus, Old Age Consultation Clinics, colleges and universities, and at the Human Engineering Laboratories which have been established in at least eight different cities in the United States by Dr. Johnson O'Connor. Valuable at any age, such tests are doubly valuable in the second half of life, to indicate which abilities are retained, which are declining, which are on the upgrade. Not infrequently, they point to hitherto unsuspected aptitudes which, trained and adapted, can open up new and exciting vistas of accomplishment.

Whatever your activities are, do not consider them mere hobbies, something you dabble at. Work at them; earn money at them if possible (if you do not need the money you can give it to your favorite charity). Even if you do something only for relaxation, let it be constructive, something with meaning and purpose; something done not just to pass the time, but because you cannot keep away from it. "Do what you love to do," said the great philosopher, Thoreau. This is sound, practical advice and sound philosophy, for the thing you love to do is the thing you will do successfully and well.

BALANCE YOUR EMOTIONS

Congenial work generates physical energy. It also generates emotional energy. You need strong, well-balanced emotions in the second half of life. You need a strong emotional drive.

In youth, emotional energy "just happens." Love for parents and teachers makes the child work hard in school. Love for families and dependents, fame, power, success—these generate young emotional drive. In the second half of life, to maintain strong, well-balanced emotions, you must fall in love with life all over again.

Fall in love again with your marriage partner, if you have one. If you are not married, why not now? Statistics prove that married people live longer than single ones. They have better-balanced emotions. They live more regular, better-balanced lives. (Also, they eat more regular, better-balanced meals.) In many ways, marriage in middle years has advantages over young marriage; it is a blend of romance and friendship, more realistic, less stormy; it presents fewer financial and vocational problems. I am not speaking of December–May marriages which, with rare exceptions, are doomed to failure from the start, but of marriages between contemporaries. Some of the most successful marriages I know of have taken place between couples in their sixties and seventies.

BALANCE YOUR MARRIAGE

Let your marriage, if any, be a sharing of mutual interests, mutual accomplishments, as well as mutual affection. Let it strike a true balance of give and take. Now is the time for a husband to turn domestic, if he wants to. In one highly delightful household of my acquaintance, the husband (retired vice-president of a textile company) does all the marketing and cooking. He has become famous for his modernly prepared meals and all their friends are eager to be invited to dinner. His wife never liked cooking, and nowadays she is too busy. She has learned hand-loom weaving, has air-conditioned the attic, and is doing a thriving textile business of her own.

A marriage that refuses to grow old is an adventurous one, not bothered by tradition, not concerned about "what will people say?" Such a marriage can exemplify, in itself, all the special charms and advantages of the second half of life.

The first "must" for a well-balanced marriage is, of course, good health. Sound nutrition, regular checkups, plenty of sleep, exercise, and rest.

The second "must" is good grooming. Carelessness in personal habits can wreck marriage, at any age; in later years it is inexcusable.

The third "must" is mental grooming. Married people learn to know each other's minds, anticipate questions, reactions, complaints. It is only fair to change and freshen your mind, keep the thoughts as well as the complexion bright and youthful.

The fourth "must" is forget your children. They are grown up now. Forget that they are your children and think of them as adults and friends. Give them love, a helping hand, advice when they ask for it. But live your own separate, individual lives.

The fifth "must" is a very important one: keep your sense of humor. If you do not have a good one, develop it. A marriage seasoned with laughter, enriched by mature humor, can never grow stale.

BALANCE YOUR FRIENDS

If you are not married, never rule out the possibility. Never shut the door on romance. Make it your habit to balance your friendships between members of your own and the opposite sex. Love your friends of both sexes. Too often, older people think the time for warmly expressed love has passed; they tend to be embarrassed even by the word "love." Love your old friends. Continually make new ones. "A man, sir," said Samuel Johnson "must keep his friendships in good repair."

Balance your friendships, also, among all generations. If you have neither children nor grandchildren, "adopt" somebody else's for your friends. Give your life roots in the growing and developing lives of young people and children. The emotional energy so generated will expand and project itself so that you find yourself loving all young people and all children, using your experience, knowledge and skills to make their world a better place than the one you have known.

Love your fellow man, whoever he is, wherever he is. As my friend Dr. Adolphe Linke says in his excellent book *A Study in Reconstructive Mental Hygiene,* "It is in profound and instinctive union with the stream of life that the greatest joy is to be found." If you feel yourself a citizen of the world, feel your own good deeply involved with the good of your fellow man, you will always be eager, interested, expectant.

BALANCE YOUR RECREATION

In the second half of life, the well-balanced person is neither a recluse nor a gadder, but something of both. He spends his leisure alone when he wants to; when he does not, he telephones a friend and makes a date or gives a party.

I am enthusiastic about the reports coming in from all over the United States of recreation clubs and groups being organized by older people—walking clubs, choral groups, folk dancing and ballroom dancing. I am particularly enthusiastic about the revival of interest in dancing for the second half of life. "To dance," Havelock Ellis tells us, "is to take part in the cosmic control of the world."

Reports from the best public ballrooms of New York, Chicago, Hollywood and other cities show that 70 percent of the clientele is over the age of 45. According to the magazine *Best Years*, the two largest national dancing school chains (Arthur Murray and Fred Astaire) report not only a majority of students between 45 and 55, but many enthusiastic clients in the seventies, eighties and nineties.

From Fred Astaire's New York studio comes the story of a highly nervous widow, in her fifties, and looking much older, who enrolled for dancing instruction on her doctor's orders. A top male instructor was assigned to her.

"You look charming and very happy," a studio executive told her truthfully, some weeks later.

"I am happy," she smiled. "I'm in love."

The executive's heart sank. It sometimes happens that pupils become overfond of their dancing instructors.

But this lady was not one of them. She added blithely, "Yes, I'm going to marry my doctor!"

BALANCE YOUR BUDGET

No Look Younger, Live Longer program could be complete if it did not include balancing the budget. Balanced diet, balanced living, balanced planning are impossible if the budget is off-base.

I know that as we have gone along you have been saying to yourself, "This man is impractical. He says, 'Get the best doctor available. Supplement your diet with vitamins and minerals. Consult a good skin specialist. Buy good shoes, well-cut clothes. Go to the best barber shop or beauty parlor you can find. Take piano lessons. Take dancing lessons.' How are everyday, average citizens of 60, 70, 80, to afford such things and still be solvent at 100?"

Actually, the Look Younger, Live Longer program is both practical and realistic. It does not suggest that you spend more money in the second half of life. It suggests, simply, that you spend your money differently.

It suggests, for instance, that you spend money for body-building foods and dietary supplements instead of for foodless chocolates, martinis, and whipped cream. That you invest several hundred dollars in a set of perfectly fitted dentures instead of an expensive intestinal operation made necessary by badly chewed food. It suggests good walking shoes, instead of taxi and bus fares. Dancing lessons now, instead of wheelchairs later on. Calcium tablets instead of chain-smoking. Adult education courses instead of bad movies. Plastic surgery instead of nervous breakdowns which drain the resources of money, time and health.

Furthermore, work is a "must" in the Look Younger, Live Longer program. The idea that a person is "retired" at 65 or thereabouts is as passé, in our modern plan of living, as a mincing gait for women and bay windows for men. *"Il faut travailler,"* repeated the great scientist, Pasteur, throughout his life. "It is necessary to work." As long ago as 172 A.D., Galen wrote, "Employment is nature's best physician and is essential to human happiness."

For the entire span of your long life you need the opportunity to be functioning and effective. Also, you need incentive. You need reward for your efforts. Spiritual rewards? Intangible rewards? Assuredly. But why not tangible rewards, too, in the form of dollars and cents?

We need jobs for the second half of life.

How are we to get these jobs?

By creating them for ourselves.

XIII. LOOK YOUNGER, LIVE LONGER GOALS

I HAVE SAID that this is no mere book that you have in your hands, that it is a passport to a new way of living, an adventure, a journey of discovery. I have told you that whatever your age, you—the person sitting there reading—you are young, you can live *and be wholly alive* longer than you ever dreamed that you could. You are a Person—V.I.P., as they say in the U.S. Armed Services—a Very Important Person.

Why?

Because there are millions of you. Today, 40,000,000 people in the United States are over 45; 18,000,000 people have passed the age of 60, 2,000,000 have passed the age of 80. Public health statistics indicate that from now on the number of Americans over 60 will increase by at least 400,000 every year. The number over 70, 80 and 90 will increase proportionately.

You are also a Very Important Problem. Do you realize this? The Old Age Problem. It is your problem. You, *and only you,* can solve it. You, and only you, are old enough, wise enough, experienced enough to redefine "old age," to demonstrate agelessness, to reorganize society in mature terms, along mature lines, on a mature level.

Millions strong, you are on the march toward good health,

good looks, good lives for a mature race of mankind, a nationwide Look Younger, Live Longer movement.

What are our Look Younger, Live Longer goals? Here are some of them. As you read, sit back and be comfortable, relax your body and let your imagination strike off sparks of its own, kindle its own enthusiasm. Let your mature wisdom, your own mature knowledge and experience, show you your own particular goal.

MEDICAL CENTERS

Here is the job for the wise older general practitioners, the specialists in chronic and degenerative diseases, eye and ear specialists, research scientists—to establish "human machine shops" for geriatrics and prevention of the disabilities of old age in every city of our country. The Mayo brothers, Johns Hopkins Hospital, and others have proved that this can be done very successfully. A group of doctors, members of the Class of 1900 of the College of Physicians and Surgeons at New York's Columbia University, have organized themselves into a Committee on Longevity to study their own old-age health problems and those of their patients in their own age group. The findings of this group will be invaluable and can be made the basis of a strong, nationwide movement. My great hope is that these doctors will give nutrition the attention it deserves. Specialized work by these and other distinguished physicians will be of immense value to all Americans in the second half of life.

HEALTH PROTECTION CENTERS

Much time, thought, and money are spent on planning for the health of our pedigreed animals. Is it not high time that we stop using haphazard methods for humans, and mobilize our American efficiency for long-range health planning for ourselves, our children and their children? I am much impressed with the health-protection experiment conducted by two English physicians who set up, in the London district of Peckham, a health center with all the equipment of a modern clinic plus a modern swimming pool and gymnastic facilities for exercise and play. The reports of increased health and disease prevention are amazing. Another health-protection center is in Dornach, Switzerland, where, under the leadership of Dr. Rudolph Steiner, a group of physicians built a magnificent place called the Goetheanum, where health protection starts with the correction of the soil; where mothers while carrying their children are given scientific care including a balanced diet of 100 percent natural foods; where children are born naturally because mothers have had training very much like that which Dr. Grantly Dick Read in New Haven now gives in his clinic.

I envision such health centers as focal points of community life, social gathering places for all age groups, where each family can be examined as a biological unit, where hidden disorders can be detected and corrected before they have a chance to become chronic. I envision these centers also as opportunities for health re-education, for teaching people how to relax, how to exercise, and above all, how to eat. Such health centers will also offer golden opportunities for the teaching of simple, basic rules of mental hygiene, and surely psychosomatic medicine has convinced us that for true health protection, we need not only sound bodies but sound minds, not only physical but "mental" diet.

This is a big job for older doctors, psychiatrists, psychiatric social workers and also for nutritionists, dietitians, former champion athletes, physical education and recreation directors.

OLD AGE COUNSELING

Dr. Lillian J. Martin of California and Dr. George Lawton of New York have demonstrated the way in which universally tested principles of clinical psychology can be applied to the needs of men and women in the second half of life. I look forward to the day when every city will have its Old Age Counseling Bureau, staffed by psychologists, vocational guidance experts, aptitude testers, rehabilitation workers who already have spent a "lifetime" of work in these fields; who know the eternal resilience of the human spirit and who passionately believe, as Dr. Lawton has so well said, that "to lose interest in setting up personal goals, some distant, some near, and to give up the struggle for their achievement—this [and only this] is growing old."

New York University's "Worry Clinic" (nonprofit) is another example of what can and should be done. Men and women who are not happy in whatever work they happened into, or who want to develop other talents for the second half of life, are given scrupulously careful, objective analyses of their aptitudes and personalities. At the end of the testing, they are given practical advice on the field in which they would be happiest and most useful.

LEGISLATIVE PLANNING

Here is the job for older statesmen, legislators, lawyers, politicians, sociologists, economists, members of professional groups and unions. These are men and women who have had many years of experience in "getting things done." Theirs is the responsibility to work for broader Social Security programs, retirement planning, old age benefits that are realistic and not "crackpot," dynamic, not makeshift. According to the March of

Time, only about 7,000 business concerns now have pension plans—a mere drop in the bucket. So far as I know, only two countries, Sweden and New Zealand, have well-organized systems for social protection. This is because citizens of both countries have unusual longevity and have, in addition (or as a result, perhaps), an unusually high general cultural level.

INDUSTRIAL PLANNING

There is great need for industry to "come of age," to curtail automatic retirement of workers at a fixed birthday regardless of whether or not the power and desire for work has lessened. Here is a job for older industrial executives who not only have the interests of their contemporaries at heart, but know from experience that the older worker is just as effective a producer as the younger man. In a recent survey of 1,000 business firms, more than three-quarters of the firms reported that older men are as productive and efficient as younger men, and there is less absenteeism.

Jobs can be shifted, working hours shortened, wages and pension benefits altered as workers grow older. To keep older workers productive is today's challenge to industry. Ford and General Motors have pioneered in this; other industries are following suit. *Time* Magazine cites an interesting example, the Ithaca Gun Company, in which "A man is not considered experienced until he is past eighty."

SMALL BUSINESS OPPORTUNITIES

Have you always wanted a business of your own? Go to your public library for books on business opportunities. They are written for younger people, but what of that? Dr. George Lawton recommends one such book, *A Business of My Own*, Pos-

sibilities in Small Community Occupations and Industries, published by Community Service, Inc. Yellow Springs, Ohio. There are many others. Also, there are in your community many other such seasoned business men and women as yourself, eager and able to launch a new venture. Find them. Put an ad in the newspaper, if necessary. Remember that at 89, Dr. Lillian J. Martin, a retired schoolteacher, ran a profitable farm with four 60-year-old assistants.

JOB PLACEMENT BUREAUS

I like to think that one day there will be in every city an employment bureau with a sign on its door: No One Under Forty-Five Need Apply. That office would be staffed entirely by people of well-seasoned maturity, "retired" personnel experts and job analysts whose aim is to secure for older applicants their share in the world's work. Such employment services already are a part of many philanthropic organizations and nonprofit public welfare societies. It is my belief that in the coming years they can be operated on a sound business basis, making it their special function to develop a new repertory of ways to utilize the judgment and experience of older people.

ADULT EDUCATION

Here is a wide-open field for retired educators—to adapt and revitalize educational methods to meet the growing demand of those who believe that it is never too late to learn. Older people want to go back to school, to learn new subjects and to learn more about themselves. Dr. George Lawton's course, "Aging Successfully," which was given at Cooper Union in New York, was attended by several hundred students, half over 60, some over 80, and in some cases husbands and wives together.

TRAINING SCHOOLS AND WORKSHOPS

We need training schools in every city where older people can know the joy of rediscovering their creative selves. Edward T. Hall, founder and director of the Universal School of Handicrafts in New York, calls this rediscovery "vitamin V" in human behavior. His students refuse to grow old; the oldest ones look younger, shed symptoms of advancing age and fears of the future, and set themselves up in new business ventures. Another model enterprise is the Opportunity School in Denver, Colorado, which for many years has trained women in their sixties for new careers.

VOLUNTEER BUREAUS

War years have proved the inestimable value of volunteer workers; they are often called "our greatest unused national resource." We need training courses for older volunteer workers, especially to work with and in behalf of the handicapped. It is not enough to give money and shed tears; active work must be done if we are to have, for example, compulsory hearing tests in schools to prevent deafness and compulsory eye drills to prevent poor vision in later life. These and many similar reforms are projects of special interest to older volunteer workers. Also, older people are the logical choice to work in behalf of other older people. The Council of Social Agencies in Chicago offers training courses for volunteers who visit the aged, listen to their problems, help in countless ways. In many communities the Red Cross Chapter includes services for the aged as part of the voluntary service program.

RECREATION CENTERS AND CLUBS

Here and there around the country, isolated "straws" show which way the wind of the future is blowing. Forty-plus clubs. The Walkers' Club of New York, all of whose members are between 60 and 80. Benjamin Rose Institute in Chicago, which has pioneered in promoting a model recreational program for older people. Philadelphia is outstanding, with forty-three clubs for older people, drawing their membership from all cultural and economic levels. I am told also, of a Grandmothers' Club—a large group of amazingly young and good-looking grandmothers —who have regular get-togethers, give dances, put on shows. (Yes, they have their annual "Grandmothers' Follies.")

There will be increasing opportunities for older people to meet and make friends with others of like tastes and interests. Not just "Lonely Hearts" clubs, but active, lively groups of people gathered together to do what they most enjoy. Dancing, choral singing, discussion groups, travel clubs, vacation camps—the possibilities are boundless. Being a nutritionist, I am most interested in seeing groups form for the congenial purpose of eating together—Eaters Anonymous Clubs of reformed overeaters, who help one another to follow the Look Younger, Live Longer dietary program. Why not start such a club in your city? It takes only one capable man or woman to do it. Already there are enthusiastic Eaters Anonymous Clubs in Detroit, Milwaukee, and Los Angeles; their numbers are increasing rapidly.

HOUSING

Growing awareness of the housing problems presented by our increasingly older population is indicated in projects developing in different parts of the country, especially in mild climates. It is my belief that coming generations of men and women in the second half of life will prefer to live with their contemporaries rather than with married children, and that the ideal arrangement will be self-managed, co-operative housing developments, apartments, and residence clubs.

Let us forever banish the concept of Homes for the Aged and think constructively, from now on, in terms of homes for the aged. Such projects would include resident doctors and nurses, recreational facilities, workshops; they would have co-operative dining rooms where, instead of dreary Old-Ladies'-Home dishes, vital, living, delicious foods will be served, "organically grown" vegetables straight from their own gardens, fresh or short-cooked.

St. Petersburg, Florida, is noted for its "planned living" for older people; some 60,000 have made it their home. Moosehaven, in Orange Park, Florida, has co-operative residence clubs and apartments especially adapted to the needs of oldsters. Another interesting project is the Colony Club for Older People in Roosevelt Park, Millville, New Jersey, which offers residents individual cottages at low rentals. There are others in California and elsewhere.

Here is a job to quicken the imagination of every architect, city planner, decorator, furniture designer, gadgeteer, dietitian and home economics expert in the second half of life—to visualize and create the living quarters they themselves want, in terms of millions of their contemporaries. The proposal of Dr. Martin Gumpert that small villages be built in Southern states, planned for the social, physical, and educational requirements of older people (why not financed by insurance companies?), is a forward step in the right direction.

PUBLIC RELATIONS

At the present time, America has gone "youth crazy." We hear of young presidents, young executives, young actors, young singers. Why do we not hear more about the tried and true mature people?

We need to work vigorously to restore the prestige of age and to break down existing social and economic prejudice against older people, in the American way, by means of planned, intelligent, long-range public relations. There is work to be done, changing existing ideas of what constitutes the useful span of life; there is work to be done to convince newspaper editors, advertising directors, and entertainment entrepreneurs that people who have lived many decades are neither marvels nor freaks but mature human beings with talent, dignity, importance, and buying power.

Here is a job for writers, artists, publicity experts, lecturers, fashion designers, entertainers in the second half of life: to re-create America's mental concept of age. It is also the individual job of every man and woman over the age of fifty to demonstrate by example that the second half of life can be the best half. Dr. George Lawton has said, "We are as young as society says we are." It is up to *you* to re-educate society.

LIVE LONGER RESTAURANTS

When, in a recent shipboard interview, I criticized American restaurants, only one national magazine, *Newsweek,* had the courage to print that criticism. But, as a pioneer in sound nutrition, I am vitally interested in America's diet. And, frankly, it seems to me that with a few exceptions the food in our restaurants from coast to coast is a disgrace. We have strict standards for the quality of liquor; why not strict standards for the quality of foods? Is it too much to hope for, that one day restaurateurs will be fined for serving foodless food?

Already there are some evidences that the doctrines I have been teaching for thirty years are being applied. Here and there, especially in larger cities, are restaurants serving good, fresh, living foods; some have "bars" serving my vegetable juice cocktails. Such restaurants do a thriving business, but there are not nearly enough of them.

Here is an opportunity for thousands of retired teachers, dietitians, and housewives who are experienced in dealing with food and with people. (It is also an opportunity for retired restaurateurs to expiate their sins.) Open Look Younger, Live Longer restaurants. If necessary, take a course in tea room management. When you have learned the mechanics, throw out the white flour, the white sugar, the hot spices, the cheap fats. In their places use whole wheat flour, molasses and honey, vegetable salt, fragrant herbs, vegetable oils and butter. Get the heaviest and shiniest stainless steel cooking utensils money can buy and make your cook (who should be mature and honest) hold up the right hand and swear never to overcook, always to short-cook foods. Serving such food will give great personal satisfaction. Moreover, intelligent people will flock to such restaurants and, knowing that there is no such thing as cheap good food, will gladly pay a fair price.

I look forward to the day when there will be Look Younger, Live Longer restaurants and bars everywhere. I hope that, in addition to their good food, their interiors will be attractive and conducive to relaxation. Use greens, yellows, and soft blues. Or use Lady Mendl's favorite color scheme—warm, dark-green walls with white trim and mirrors, and more mirrors.

Above all, I hope that these restaurants will never be faddish or "culty." We are not faddists or cultists in the Look Younger, Live Longer program. With us, correct eating is not an obsession. It is fun. We do not chew nuts and grimly munch raw vegetables as did fanatic members of the late and unlamented Nut and Berry Club, which fortunately put itself out of business. We eat well-balanced, well-cooked and delicious foods and enjoy it. So far am I from being a faddist, that I believe the time will come when Look Younger, Live Longer menus will be served not only in special restaurants but in all restaurants, when they will be considered the modern menus of the modern age.

LIVE LONGER FOOD SHOPS

Large chain stores do not sell 100 percent whole wheat flour and cereals, whole corn meal, untreated natural sugar and molasses, because these foods do not keep indefinitely in storage, as do the refined products. Unrefined foods must be fresh. Some health food shops have small mills where all whole cereals are freshly ground. Because the incomparable goodness of such 100 percent foods is being more and more widely realized, health food shops are springing up everywhere. But there is room for thousands more. If you like and understand just two subjects—food and people—a health food shop can be an exciting as well as a profitable adventure for the second half of your life. But do make it an attractive, good-health food shop, not one of those dreary little ill-health food places.

Teachers, doctors' wives, ministers' wives, nurses, YWCA workers are especially well adapted to this sort of project. Man and wife combinations are ideal—one can do the counseling and selling, the other the buying and ordering. Many other specialty foods that cannot be obtained in regular stores are sold in health food shops. Such natural foods as uncooked honey, unsulphured blackstrap molasses, unsprayed dried fruits, fresh wheat germ, wheat germ oil, brewers' yeast, iodized vegetable salt, powdered milk, soya bean flour, peanut flour—staples which sooner or later will be used by all intelligent people. Correctly balanced vitamin and mineral products and calcium tablets have immense sales in these shops; a health bar serving fresh vegetable and fruit juices is an added attraction. Such miracle drinks as my "milk lassie" and other delicious fortified beverages constantly attract new clients. Think it over. Are you one of the people especially equipped to run a Live Longer food shop?

LOOK YOUNGER BEAUTY SHOPS

Some years ago, when I wrote my book, *Eat and Grow Beautiful,* I expressed the hope that in time my inside-and-outside plan would be incorporated by some of our smart New York and Beverly Hills beauty salons. I had not long to wait. Elizabeth Arden established her beauty farm in Maine. In New York, Dorothy Gray engaged one of my assistants and opened a beauty bar. Helena Rubenstein opened a "food for beauty" restaurant, and Ann Delafield (formerly at Arden's) set up her famous and profitable Success School at Richard Hudnut's.

So far, so good. But this is only the beginning. Americans are beauty-conscious. American women are by nature the most beautiful women in the world; the mixture of our nationalities, diets, and clothes all help. American women in the second half of life already are learning to give more, rather than less, attention to grooming and appearance.

I look forward to the day when in every city there will be Look Younger beauty shops that cater especially to the mature woman.

Such shops will give scientific beauty treatments in the Body Slant position to improve circulation in our scalps and faces. They will serve fortified milk drinks and fresh vegetable juice cocktails—enrichment for the blood stream, bringing beauty from within.

Such shops will be run by mature beauty operators who understand the special needs of adult American women and have special interest in teaching them the art and science of agelessness. Here will develop new fashions in smart and conservative hair-dos, in dignified and natural make-up. Already, Beautymasters of Beverly Hills, California, is instructing its women representatives according to a co-ordinated beauty plan. After thorough training in diet, exercise, reducing, hair care, eye care, make-up, and the art of relaxation, these representatives are taught to present this plan in the privacy of the client's home. Anyone who is interested in such a career can write to them directly.

Here is a business with a future. Teaching others the art of youthfulness is a good way to keep youthful oneself. And beauty is a profession which knows no depression.

ORGANIC GARDENING

The idea of organic gardening is new to most Americans, but in England thousands of people have learned to produce superior fruits and vegetables even on small plots of land. And wherever a family had an organic garden, their health and well-being greatly increased.

Here are three good reasons for taking up organic gardening: first, to produce more delicious and nutritious foods for yourself, your family and friends; second, to avoid foods treated with harmful fertilizers and insecticides; third, to provide yourself a fascinating new occupation which may possibly become a source of income as well.

Organic gardening is not difficult, once you have learned to let the enzymes of compost and the earthworms do most of the work for you. Earthworms do your plowing. Under light mulches, soil becomes soft and crumbly, making spading and hoeing scarcely necessary. Your mulches smother out weeds. If you feel like working in your garden, you do so. If you prefer to relax and watch its progress, you can let your garden largely take care of itself.

While health can certainly be improved by selecting for nutritive value such foods as are available, nevertheless, owing to our soil depletion, many of our garden products today lack the vitamins, minerals, and other nutrients they should contain.

Commercial fertilizers supplying phosphorus, nitrogen, and potassium force the growth of vegetables, but fail to furnish seventeen or more other nutrients needed by healthy plants. As these plants are deficient in the missing nutrients, the animals and humans living on such plant foods likewise suffer deficiencies. This chain reaction has resulted in a tremendous increase in diseases among plants, animals, and humans alike and is exactly the reason why we must fortify our present diets with the vitamins and minerals we *should* but do not get from our foods, grown in deficient soil.

The *Journal of the American Medical Association* recently pointed out that more than 7,000 insecticides now being used for farming purposes are as poisonous to humans as to insects. These harmful substances also kill millions of valuable insects needed to combat the crop-destroying ones. Cases of poisoning from sprays left on vegetables are becoming more frequent, and for those with sensitive digestions, I recommend washing sprayed vegetables and fruits in the formula on page 331.

When foods are grown organically, however, not only is their vitamin, mineral, and protein content greatly increased, but their flavor is incredibly superior to that of foods grown on chemically fertilized soil. It has been proved beyond doubt by the proponents of organic gardening that healthier plants can be grown; that diseases of plants can be corrected by rebuilding the soil and revitalizing it with natural humus; and that sprays and poisons become unnecessary. And persons who have eaten only organically grown foods for a number of years find marked improvement in their health.

You will find organic gardening one of the most exciting and satisfying of occupations. You may start reading up on the subject with mild interest, find that interest mounting with each new discovery, vow you'll not become fanatic on the subject—and quickly become just that.

Browsing through some of the books would surely whet anyone's appetite for gardening. *Harnessing the Earthworm,* by Dr. Thomas J. Barrett, is a fascinating account of how the Nile Valley has sustained the richest soil in the world, even though it has been under constant cultivation for a known span of 6,000 years.

Have you read *Pleasant Valley* and *Malabar Farm,* by Louis Bromfield? Strictly speaking, Bromfield is not an organic gardener, but he can make almost anyone want to buy a farm.

I also recommend Edward H. Faulkner's books, *Plowman's Folly, Uneasy Money,* and *A Second Look.* While you may not agree with all of his arguments, you will surely acquire a great respect for the moisture-holding power of organic material stirred into the soil.

Farmers of Forty Centuries, by F. H. King, and all of the writings of Dr. Ehrenfried Pfeiffer, as well as those of Sir Albert Howard and his wife, Louise E. Howard, also are valuable. *Compost Making by the Quick Return Method,* by Mary E. Bruce, and *Compost and How To Make It,* by J. E. Rodale, will also give you hours of interesting reading and inspiration. You can keep up with all that is new in diet, health, and organic gardening by subscribing to *Diet Digest,* published at 100 Stevens Avenue, Mount Vernon, New York.

And now, as you reach the final page of this book, are you saying to yourself, "I am at the end of this journey called *Look Younger, Live Longer?*"

I hope that you are not. I hope that, instead, you are saying to yourself, "My journey is just beginning. It is a journey that will continue for the rest of my long life." As I write these lines, I am in Italy. Before me lies the blue, blue Mediterranean. On my right towers Mount Aetna, covered with eternal snow. The morning breeze brings me the fragrance of thousands of flowers in my garden. I am at peace, deeply grateful to the Master Chemist that I am a small part of this radiant and beautiful world. I am "all right."

This is really the *summum bonum.* Not money nor culture nor fame; those are mere accessories. The greatest good is this feeling of "all rightness," of being in harmony with oneself, with nature, united with the great stream of life.

Come along with me. Join me in my never-ceasing wonder and admiration for the most marvelous instrument ever created—the self-healing, self-renewing human body. Join me in my crusade to give your body—all human bodies, everywhere—the good food, utter relaxation, and wise understanding that they need to remain youthful, vigorous, and buoyant for at least one hundred years.

Here is our world, the Look Younger, Live Longer world. Here is our job—to help shape this world on Look Younger, Live Longer principles.

Whatever you choose as your particular job for the second half of your life, good luck to you. Good health to you. Good looks. Long life.

Good living!

Casa Cuseni
Taormina, Sicily
Italy

LOOK YOUNGER, LIVE LONGER
DIET PLAN

EMEMBER for the rest of your long life to include in your diet more proteins, more vitamins, more minerals, less starch and sugar (and never the refined), and as little fat as possible. Whenever possible, eat your salad first; if mastication is a problem, have a liquid salad.

If you have a stubborn wife or stupid cook, fortify your own meals. Have a good-looking special tray with a jar of dry brewers' yeast, powdered milk, wheat germ, your vitamins, your minerals, blackstrap molasses, honey, vegetable salt (iodized), your favorite spices; and you can go blithely on your happy way, independent of all.

BREAKFAST: Your choice of: fruit or fruit juice, preferably fresh. ALSO your choice of: any natural cereal with milk (not cream), or waffles or muffins, all fortified with one or two table-spoons of wheat germ; or eggs, any way but fried, with whole wheat toast. ALSO your choice of: café au lait (hot milk and coffee, half and half), milk or fortified milk drink. PLUS YOUR LIVE LONGER RITUAL: Make it a daily habit to fortify yourself for the whole day with 1 fish liver oil capsule for your vitamins A and D, 1 100-milli-gram tablet of ascorbic acid for your vitamin C, and 1 30-milligram capsule of wheat germ oil for your vitamin E; or obtain from your nutritionist a balanced vitamin formula containing all these.

MIDMORNING: Your choice of: fruit drink or milk drink, fortified with 1 tablespoon of brewers' yeast or powdered skim milk or both; or a glass of yogurt fortified with molasses.

LUNCH: Your choice of: eggs, if none for breakfast; or cheese, or meat, or fortified cream soup. ALSO your choice of: vegetables and fruits. ALSO your choice of: whole wheat, or rye bread. ALSO your choice of: beverage: milk, yogurt, buttermilk, or fortified milk drink.

MIDAFTERNOON: Your choice of: milk drink or fruit drink, fortified with powdered milk or brewers' yeast; or yogurt fortified with molasses.

DINNER: Your choice of: soup or vegetable juice cocktail (liquid salads), fortified with brewers' yeast. ALSO your choice of: lean meat, or fish, or fowl, or cheese, or soya beans. ALSO your choice of: one dark-green or yellow vegetable and one raw salad with fortified salad dressing. ALSO, if not overweight, one whole potato or one helping of brown rice, or buckwheat, or gluten spaghetti. ALSO your choice of: dessert: fresh or stewed fruit à la Lady Mendl, or yogurt with fruit, or, occasionally, open-faced Vienna Pie. ALSO your choice of: beverage: demitasse or New Orleans cup (if your doctor has forbidden coffee), or fortified milk.

BEFORE RETIRING: Your choice of: fortified hot or cold milk, or fruit juice fortified with yeast, or yogurt fortified with honey and molasses.

And here are one week's LIVE LONGER MENUS to give you concrete examples of how easily your meals may be planned:

BREAKFAST:
  Orange juice, large glass
  Poached egg on whole wheat toast
  Café au lait or fortified milk drink

  Your daily Live Longer Ritual: Fortify yourself with 1 vitamin A and D capsule, 1 vitamin C tablet (100 milligrams), 1 vitamin E capsule (30 milligrams), and 2 mineral tablets containing calcium, phosphorus, and a trace of iodine. Drink down with breakfast beverage.

MIDMORNING: Fortified fruit or milk drink; or yogurt with molasses and honey.

LUNCH: Grilled cheese sandwich on wheat germ bread
One glass of yogurt, buttermilk or café au lait

MIDAFTERNOON: Your choice as midmorning

DINNER: Grapefruit and avocado salad with fortified lemon oil dressing
Broiled hamburgers with parsley and wheat germ
Fortified potatoes
Fresh or frozen peas with herbs
Yogurt sprinkled with honey and grated orange rind
Demitasse (small black coffee)

BEDTIME: Fortified milk drink, hot or cold; with it drink down 2 calcium tablets.

Good night, happy dreams! Remember, what you ate today, walks and talks tomorrow.

BREAKFAST: Apple juice, large glass
Hot cakes fortified with powdered milk and wheat germ and served with honey
Café au lait or fortified milk drink

Your daily Live Longer Ritual: Fortify yourself with 1 vitamin A and D capsule, 1 vitamin C tablet (100 milligrams), 1 vitamin E capsule (30 milligrams), and 2 mineral tablets containing calcium, phosphorus, and a trace of iodine. Drink down with breakfast beverage.

MIDMORNING: Fortified fruit or milk drink, or yogurt with molasses and honey

LUNCH: Large dish of cottage cheese with shredded carrots
Rye bread toast
Café au lait or milk drink

MIDAFTERNOON: Your choice as midmorning

DINNER: Salad bowl or hot broth
Broiled calves' liver
String beans with herbs
Parsleyed potatoes
Custard fortified with powdered milk, served with honeyed fruit
Demitasse (small black coffee)

BEDTIME: Fortified milk drink, hot or cold; with it drink down 2 calcium tablets.

Good night, happy dreams! Remember, what you ate today, walks and talks tomorrow.

BREAKFAST: Sliced bananas sprinkled with honey and wheat germ and served with milk
Scrambled eggs
Wheat germ muffins with honey
Café au lait or fortified milk drink

Your daily Live Longer Ritual: Fortify yourself with 1 vitamin A and D capsule, 1 vitamin C tablet (100 milligrams), 1 vitamin E capsule (30 milligrams), and 2 mineral tablets containing calcium, phosphorus, and a trace of iodine.

MIDMORNING: Fortified fruit or milk drink, or yogurt with molasses and honey

LUNCH: Cold cuts (lean)
                    Salad of tomatoes, cucumbers, and celery
                        with yogurt dressing
                    Buttermilk, tea, or café au lait

MIDAFTERNOON: Your choice as midmorning

DINNER: Salad bowl or liquid salad
                    Meat balls fortified with powdered milk and
                        wheat germ
                    Shredded short-cooked beets
                    Yogurt with fresh or frozen raspberries
                    Demitasse (small black coffee)

BEDTIME: Fortified milk drink, hot or cold; with it
                    drink down 2 calcium tablets.

Good night, happy dreams! Remember, what you ate today,
walks and talks tomorrow.

BREAKFAST: One-half grapefruit
                    Whole wheat cereal cooked 5 minutes and
                        served with milk and honey
                    Café au lait or fortified milk drink

                    Your daily Live Longer Ritual: Fortify your-
                        self with 1 vitamin A and D capsule, 1
                        vitamin C tablet (100 milligrams), 1 vita-
                        min E capsule (30 milligrams), and 2
                        mineral tablets containing calcium, phos-
                        phorus, and a trace of iodine.

MIDMORNING: Fortified fruit or milk drink, or yogurt with
                        molasses and honey

LUNCH: Cream of asparagus soup prepared by liquefy-
                        ing green asparagus tips with fresh and
                        powdered milk
                    Whole wheat crackers
                    Café au lait or fortified milk drink

MIDAFTERNOON: Your choice as midmorning

DINNER: Tomato and avocado salad
Roast chicken
Fortified potatoes
Milk gravy fortified with powdered milk
Fresh or honeyed fruit
Demitasse (small black coffee)

BEDTIME: Fortified milk drink, hot or cold; with it
drink down 2 calcium tablets.

Good night, happy dreams! Remember, what you ate today,
walks and talks tomorrow.

BREAKFAST: Sliced orange
Boiled egg cooked until yolk is well jellied
Whole wheat toast with honey
Café au lait or fortified milk drink

Your daily Live Longer Ritual: Fortify yourself with 1 vitamin A and D capsule, 1
vitamin C tablet (100 milligrams), 1 vitamin E capsule (30 milligrams), and 2
mineral tablets containing calcium, phosphorus, and a trace of iodine.

MIDMORNING: Fortified fruit or milk drink, or yogurt with
molasses and honey

LUNCH: Cheese soufflé
Creamed spinach
Sliced pineapple
Café au lait, fortified milk drink, or tea

MIDAFTERNOON: Your choice as midmorning

DINNER: Clam chowder made with fresh and pow-
dered milk
Broiled lean fish
Fortified potatoes

Zucchini squash or spinach
Fruit compote à la Lady Mendl
Demitasse (small black coffee)

BEDTIME: Fortified milk drink, hot or cold; with it
drink down 2 calcium tablets.

Good night, happy dreams! Remember, what you ate today,
walks and talks tomorrow.

BREAKFAST: Cantaloupe sprinkled with wheat germ and
honey
Shredded wheat
Crisp, drained bacon
Café au lait or fortified milk drink

Your daily Live Longer Ritual: Fortify yourself with 1 vitamin A and D capsule, 1
vitamin C tablet (100 milligrams), 1 vitamin E capsule (30 milligrams), and 2
mineral tablets containing calcium, phosphorus, and a trace of iodine.

MIDMORNING: Fortified fruit or milk drink, or yogurt with
molasses and honey

LUNCH: Cream of celery soup prepared in liquefier
with celery tops, onion, fresh and powdered milk
Wheat germ crackers
Café au lait, fortified milk drink, or tea

MIDAFTERNOON: Your choice as midmorning

DINNER: Gelatin salad prepared by liquefying mixed
greens in tomato juice
Meat loaf with parsley and wheat germ
Sautéed parsnips or carrots
Viennese fruit pastry
Demitasse (small black coffee)

BEDTIME: Fortified milk drink, hot or cold; with it
                       drink down 2 calcium tablets.
Good night, happy dreams! Remember, what you ate today,
walks and talks tomorrow.

BREAKFAST: Sliced peaches, fresh or frozen
                       Waffles fortified with wheat germ and served
                       with honey
                       Café au lait or fortified milk drink

                       Your daily Live Longer Ritual: Fortify your-
                       self with 1 vitamin A and D capsule, 1
                       vitamin C tablet (100 milligrams), 1 vita-
                       min E capsule (30 milligrams), and 2
                       mineral tablets containing calcium, phos-
                       phorus, and a trace of iodine.

MIDMORNING: Fortified fruit or milk drink, or yogurt with
                       molasses and honey

LUNCH: Chicken or meat salad
                       Rye bread toast
                       Yogurt with fruit
                       Café au lait or fortified milk drink

MIDAFTERNOON: Your choice as midmorning

DINNER: Salad of shredded spinach blended into cot-
                       tage cheese, served with sliced tomato on
                       lettuce
                       Salmon loaf fortified with wheat germ and
                       powdered yeast
                       Shredded short-cooked carrots
                       Caramel junket containing 1 cup powdered
                       milk to 1 pint fresh milk, sweetened to
                       taste with brown sugar
                       Demitasse (small black coffee)

BEDTIME: Fortified milk drink, hot or cold; with it drink down 2 calcium tablets.

Good night, happy dreams! Remember, what you ate today, walks and talks tomorrow.

LOOK YOUNGER RECIPES

FROM THIS DAY ON, you can make richer, tastier, and more healthful meals by fortifying your favorite dishes. In this book, it is impossible to teach you the entire art and science of cooking for health. For that I refer you to my cook book, *The Gaylord Hauser Cook Book,* a complete course in the scientific cooking of meats, vegetables, and hundreds of delicious recipes of the tastiest foods you ever ate. Here, in our Look Younger, Live Longer plan, I want to give you some unusual and different recipes, but more than anything, I want to show you how you can fortify practically all of your everyday dishes with powdered skim milk, powdered brewers' yeast, whole wheat germ and oil, molasses, honey, and yogurt.

Since most older people are deficient in protein, calcium, riboflavin, and other vitamins of the B family, powdered skim milk, which is cheap, is ideal for fortifying purposes. The chief food value of milk lies in its solids and not in the cream, especially since cream is so heavy in cholesterol. The addition of half a cup of dried powdered skim milk adds more than 34 grams of first class protein to the diet, which is equal to five eggs, and much, much cheaper. May I suggest that you be extravagant in your use of powdered skim milk. Buy the kind that comes in vacuum sealed cans, and besides making delicious milk drinks with it, use it in custards, in soups, in ice cream, in all your baking. Here are some recipes to start you:

FORTIFIED MILK AND MILK DRINKS

Fortified Milk

Pour 2 cups fresh milk into a 1-quart Mason jar and add ½ cup powdered skim milk. Shake vigorously and when smooth, add 2 more cups fresh milk. If you have an electric mixer, simply pour the powdered milk into the fresh milk and mix for 1 minute. Here you have the nourishment of 2 quarts of milk for drinking and cooking purposes. You may add honey or molasses to taste, but not chocolate because it interferes with the absorption of calcium so badly needed in the second part of life.

Milk Lassie

Beat 2 level tablespoons powdered skim milk and 2 teaspoons blackstrap molasses into a cup fresh milk. Also add 1 teaspoon powdered brewers' yeast. Beat until smooth. Serve cold between meals or hot before retiring, but do not boil.

Honey Lass

Put 1 tablespoon honey and molasses into 1 cup fortified hot milk. Stir with fork until smooth. Excellent for weight-gaining when taken between meals or before retiring.

Fortified Milk for Reducers

Most of the calories are in the cream of milk, but removing the cream from whole milk still leaves too much fat. It is therefore wise to order a quart of skim milk from your milkman and fortify this skim milk. In this manner you receive the double amount of protein, calcium, riboflavin and other vitamins of the B family, in one quart of milk. Such fortified skim milk prevents hunger pains and gives that satisfied feeling when taken with or between meals. I recommend this fortified milk drink to all Eaters Anonymous as their best friend. Drink a quart a day, use it for cooking, and make delicious fat-free yogurt with it. Here is how to make this super food so that you won't even know it is skimmed milk:

Put a little less than a quart of fresh skim milk into a Mason jar or electric mixer and add a scant half-cup of dried skim milk. Also add 2 tablespoons dried brewers' yeast and 1 tablespoon blackstrap molasses. Shake well or mix until frothy. Keep on ice and drink to your heart's content during the day; and heat a cup to the simmering point (do not boil) and take as a nightcap for deep, sound sleep.

YOGURT MEANS LONG LIFE

Down through the ages, yogurt has played an important part. It is interesting that, regardless of the country, the word "yogurt" has the same meaning. The Armenians call yogurt *matzoon*. The Yugoslavs call it *kisselo mleko*, and King Peter assured me that there are hundreds of centenarians in his country who thrive on this *kisselo mleko*. The Russians love their yogurt with their black bread, and call it *varenetz*. The French eat quantities of yogurt with *fraises de bois*, and call it *yoghourt*. In Sardinia, they call yogurt *gioddu*, in India *dadhi*; in Egypt, it's called *lebenraib*; but it always means the same thing—*long life*.

How to Make Fortified Yogurt at Home

Making good yogurt is much like making good coffee; some do and some don't. And yet thousands of Russian, Yugoslav, and Bulgarian peasants make delicious yogurt without fuss and without thermometers. If you live in a large city, you can buy good ready-made yogurt. However, if you have a big family, it is quite expensive when you have to buy several quarts a day. Here, then, is a million-dollar secret for making your own yogurt, fortified with nourishing powdered skim milk, and no more expensive than ordinary milk. Here is the simplest procedure:

Add ½ cup powdered skim milk to 1 quart fresh milk, and shake in a Mason jar or mix in an electric mixer. Heat this mixture until it is good and hot, but do not let the milk boil. Into this hot but not boiling milk (the peasant puts a drop on the palm of the hand; it should feel hot but should not burn) you stir 3 tablespoons ready-made yogurt. Pour this mixture into a milk bottle, or a double boiler, or any utensil, and place it in warm water, near the pilot light of your stove or near a radiator. Cover it with a shawl, much the same as you would raising dough for bread-making. In about 5 hours, you will have a quart of delicious fortified yogurt. Place in refrigerator and eat it for health, for fun, and for better looks. Remember that a pint, or still better a quart of yogurt, daily, is desirable in our Look Younger program.

Such yogurt has many advantages over ordinary milk. The protein is easier to digest, the calcium is more easily assimilated by older people, and, of course, the vitamins of the valuable B family which the yogurt bacteria manufacture in the intestines are invaluable. Also, excessive gas and putrefaction, from which many mature people suffer, are gradually eliminated since the troublesome bacteria cannot live in the lactic acid of yogurt.

If you are unable to buy fresh yogurt in your city, you should write to your nearest health food store and order a bottle of yogurt culture. You might also investigate the yogurt maker, an inexpensive gadget which looks very much like a large thermos bottle, and which makes delicious yogurt while you sleep.

Fat-free Yogurt for Reducers

The laziest and most pleasant way to stop overeating is to keep the stomach (the brute) filled and contented with fat-free yogurt. Since adults often lack the enzymes to digest the sugar in milk, the calories you derive from a quart of fat-free yogurt are those of 34 grams of protein or only 136 calories per quart. By adding ½ cup of dried skim milk to the quart of fresh skim milk, you actually consume only 272 calories, but what is most important for reducers, you obtain 68 grams of first class protein to keep the muscles of face and body firm and young. The longer you reduce with this fat-free yogurt, the better for your skin, hair, and eyes, for you also obtain large amounts of the entire vitamin B family.

For making fat-free yogurt, follow the directions for making fortified yogurt, but use skim milk ordered from your dairy in place of whole milk. Remember that simply removing the cream from regular milk still leaves too much fat. Learn to enjoy the natural flavor of fat-free yogurt and you are headed for a slimmer and trimmer future. If you need additional flavor, try brewers' yeast, cinnamon, nutmeg, or a bit of blackstrap molasses, but use these additions sparingly.

Yogurt Tomato Juice

For a delicious and nutritious appetizer, mix equal amounts of tomato juice and fortified yogurt. Add a bit of vegetable salt and paprika, or a dash of your favorite sauce. Blend well and serve chilled. This delicious mixture keeps well when refrigerated, and is excellent for breakfast or as an appetizer before dinner.

I recommend this combination highly and dedicate it to Count Cassini, our Cholly Knickerbocker of New York, who is a yogurt enthusiast and who eats it frequently for breakfast.

Yogurt Fruit Cup

Put alternate layers of honeyed strawberries, sliced pineapple, and sliced bananas in shiny dessert glasses. Alternate each layer of fruit with a layer of chilled yogurt. Decorate top with a large strawberry, rolled in coarse brown sugar crystals, and listen to your guests rave.

Raspberry Yogurt

Mix 1 cup thick yogurt, ½ cup canned raspberries or ½ cup raspberry juice, and put in refrigerator. Serve in dessert glasses and sprinkle top with a bit of orange blossom honey.

Yogurt Blinchiki

Make very thin pancakes (crêpes) and spread thinly with raspberry or apricot jam. Then blend fresh cottage cheese with fortified yogurt, spread on top, and roll the pancakes up. Place them in a medium hot oven and bake for about 20 minutes. Serve hot and top each *blinchiki* with slightly honeyed yogurt. A delicious luncheon dish or dessert.

Yogurt Paprika

Have 1 pound of veal cut into cubes. Melt 2 tablespoons margarine in a heavy skillet and add 1 teaspoon mild and very red paprika. Add 2 sliced onions and sauté lightly. Salt the meat, roll in wheat germ, and place in skillet. Sauté until the meat is a delicious brown. Now whip a cup of yogurt until creamy, and pour slowly over the meat. Cover the skillet and cook slowly for another 20 minutes. Dedicated to my friend Hilda West.

FORTIFIED FRUIT DRINKS

Fruit juices are excellent sources of vitamins, especially vitamin C which helps to keep our connective tissues young; but with the addition of dried skim milk, brewers' yeast, wheat germ, and natural sweets as molasses and honey, we can make the most Lucullean and delicious drinks. Not only will these be rich in vitamin C but the vitamins of the B family, vitamin E, many minerals, and the ever-necessary amino acids are contained in the proteins of skim milk and powdered yeast. Most of these mixtures can be made in an ordinary cocktail shaker, but for superb results, you should invest in one of the electric mixers which fletcherizes everything into the consistency of smooth, easier-to-digest liquids. Be inquisitive, try all the different drinks; then experiment and create new combinations. Don't overdo, as some health faddists do, and make evil-tasting combinations that taste like alfalfa. There must be pleasure in eating; Americans eat with their eyes, so make everything as attractive and appetizing as possible. Drink these concentrated mixtures through a straw, and slowly, please. Here are some favorite combinations:

Curvaceous Cocktail

Into 1 cup orange juice or milk beat 1 egg yolk, 1 tablespoon wheat germ, and 1 teaspoon of honey.

Orange Milk Shake

Shake or mix 1 glass orange juice with 2 tablespoons powdered skim milk and 1 tablespoon honey. Mix until smooth and frothy, and drink at once for quick and added energy.

I dedicate this drink to Jessica Dragonette, beloved singing star.

Pineapple Shake

Put ¼ cup powdered skim milk and 1 teaspoon honey into a large glass of unsweetened pineapple juice. Beat until frothy. For better nourishment, also add 1 teaspoon powdered brewers' yeast, and increase to 1 heaping tablespoon as you become accustomed to the flavor. Also try this combination with grape juice, loganberry juice, apricot juice, apple juice (canned or frozen).

All-in-One Cocktail

Pour a glass of pineapple juice or apple juice into an electric mixer. Add 1 tablespoon nut kernels, 1 teaspoon wheat germ, 1 teaspoon powdered brewers' yeast, and 1 teaspoon honey. For extra flavor, add 1 tablespoon of berries or a few slices of banana. Mix thoroughly, and in a minute's time you have a most delicious "building drink." Sip it through a straw—a meal in one glass.

This combination I dedicate to Leopold Stokowski, who years ago learned about the importance of nutrition.

Pineapple Delight

Pour 1 cup unsweetened pineapple juice into an electric mixer. Add 2 tablespoons wheat germ, 1 tablespoon powdered skim milk, and 1 teaspoon honey or molasses. Mix until smooth and creamy, and serve at once.

Banana Milk Shake

Mix in an electric mixer 1 very ripe banana, 2 tablespoons powdered skim milk, 1 teaspoon honey, and 1 glass unsweetened pineapple juice.

Banana Cream Shake

One very ripe banana, 1 tablespoon dried skim milk, 1 teaspoon dried brewers' yeast, 1 teaspoon blackstrap molasses or honey, and 1 cup fresh milk are thoroughly mixed in an electric mixer for about 30 seconds, or until smooth, creamy, and delicious.

I dedicate this drink to the lovely Barbara Hutton Troubetzkoy.

FORTIFIED DRINKS FOR REDUCERS

Mix ½ cup dried skim milk with 1 quart fresh skim milk. For additional flavor, add not more than 2 teaspoons blackstrap molasses, and a pinch of vegetable salt. Shake in Mason jar until smooth or put in electric mixer until frothy and delicious. Keep in refrigerator and drink a quart a day.

Mix 4 tablespoons dried brewers' yeast (celery flavor) with 1 quart canned tomato juice. For additional flavor, add ½ teaspoon vegetable salt, 1 tablespoon lemon juice, and your choice of a tablespoon of parsley or chives or green onion, or a teaspoon of caraway seeds. Shake in Mason jar or whip until frothy, and keep in refrigerator. Excellent when taken just before meals as an appetizer.

Mix 1 pint tomato juice, 1 pint sauerkraut juice, 4 tablespoons dried brewers' yeast, plus a pinch of caraway seeds, and keep in refrigerator.

Mix 1 pint tomato juice, 1 pint fat-free yogurt, a dash of vegetable salt and 2 tablespoons dried brewers' yeast. Shake in Mason jar or in electric mixer until smooth, and keep in refrigerator. Excellent for breakfast in place of plain juices.

Mix 1 teaspoon dried brewers' yeast (preferably celery flavor), a bit of chopped parsley and a pinch of vegetable salt into a glass of canned mixed vegetable juice.

Mix 1 glass of sauerkraut juice, a pinch of caraway seeds, and 1 teaspoon dried brewers' yeast in electric mixer until smooth.

Mix ½ glass tomato juice with ½ glass sauerkraut juice and add 1 teaspoon dried brewers' yeast.

Mix ½ glass fat-free yogurt with ½ glass tomato juice and 1 teaspoon dried brewers' yeast.

Mix 1 teaspoon dried brewers' yeast into a glass of grapefruit juice.

Mix 1 teaspoon dried brewers' yeast into a cup of leftover vegetable water or Hauser Broth.

Note: Since dried brewers' yeast is such a wonder food, try to increase the amount to a tablespoonful.

LIVER TONIC AND COOKED LIVER

Liver Tonic

The less you cook liver, the more healthful for anemic, run-down people. However, the eating of raw, or almost raw, liver was a hardship until the invention of the electric gadget which fletcherizes raw liver so finely that the unpalatable taste is entirely eliminated.

I recommend this drink especially to those people who need nourishment quickly and in concentrated form. Such a liver tonic should be served in all homes for the aged. Here is the recipe:

Put 1 cup vegetable broth or any vegetable juice into an electric mixer and add 1 tablespoon fresh parsley and 1 slice onion. Mix until smooth. Now add 1 tablespoon very fresh raw liver and mix another half minute. Season with a bit of vegetable salt and drink at once. There will be no taste of liver, and the improvement brought about by taking one glass a day for two weeks will amaze you.

Not only liver, but heart, sweetbreads, kidney, and other glandular organs which are sometimes ordered by physicians, can be made palatable in this manner. Raw organ meats are becoming more and more popular because they are unusually rich in vitamins, hormones, and as yet undiscovered important substances.

Liver de Luxe

Have calves' liver cut in thin noodle-like strips. Put 1 tablespoon butter or peanut oil in heavy skillet, and in it sauté 1 sliced onion and 1 tablespoon wheat germ. When onion and wheat germ turn golden brown, add strips of liver and sauté for another 3 minutes. Sprinkle with ½ teaspoon vegetable salt. To tenderize liver, cover skillet for 1 minute before removing from fire. Serve this liver twice a week.

Broiled Liver

Brush sliced liver with peanut oil and sprinkle with vegetable salt. Place on oiled broiler and broil not longer than 3 minutes on each side. Place on hot plate, dot with butter, and sprinkle with chopped parsley or green onions.

Sautéed Liver

Roll half-inch thick slices of liver in wheat germ. Melt butter or margarine in iron skillet. Sauté liver slices about 3 minutes on each side, or until golden brown. Serve with onions or apples, or, for variety's sake, add yogurt to liver and let simmer for 5 minutes. Sprinkle with chives or green onions.

DELICIOUS BREAD, MUFFINS, CEREALS, ETC.

Before you make any of these baked foods, you should study the analysis of the different flours and the five wonder foods. Notice the difference between the popular white flour and the natural whole wheat flour. Notice the richness of the humble and despised dried skim milk; one-half cup contains 53 grams of first class protein (almost sufficient protein for the whole day). Notice the calcium and the niacin content, all so necessary for our Look Younger Recipes. Notice that one tablespoon of powdered brewers' yeast fortifies with 4 grams of protein and gives you all those B vitamins for your nerves and the "inner man." And look at all the calcium, plus all the B vitamins and iron, that one tablespoon of blackstrap molasses furnishes, compared with the nothingness of white syrup (white sugar contains even less). And finally, notice the magnificent food content of a half-cup of soya flour, which is easily obtainable everywhere; and peanut flour, which I hope will soon be in all the good health shops.

Swear, now, that for the rest of your long life you will use these foods; that you will fortify your diet with these foods whenever possible; that you will use less baking powder and more brewers' yeast in your baking; that you will use wheat germ in your morning cereal, in your baking, and in your salad bowl; that you will make blackstrap molasses, from the deep south, your favorite sweetener; and that you will each and every day use half a cup of dried skim milk in the form of delicious and fortified milk drinks. As a result, Dr. H. C. Sherman of Columbia University promises "the preservation of the characteristics of youth," which means abundant vitality, a clear skin, and a natural enthusiasm for life.

Fortify Your Own Bread

Here is a delicious high-protein bread, very easy to make. Such a loaf could give pleasure and nourishment to a small family for a whole week. Combine in a large bowl 2½ cups whole wheat

JUDGE THE VALUE OF THESE FOODS FOR YOURSELF

	Grams Protein	Calcium	Iron	Vit. B₁	Vit. B₂	Niacin
1 cup whole wheat flour	12	45	5.0	0.48	0.16	5.5
1 cup best white flour	10	20	1.0	0.08	0.03	0.8
1 cup soya flour	37	200	7.4	0.65	0.37	8.2
1 cup peanut flour	59	65	10.0	0.6	0.3	18.9
½ cup wheat germ	24	750	7.5	2.60	0.75	24.2
½ cup skim milk dry	53	1930	1.9	0.55	2.61	19.2
½ cup fresh milk whole	4	150	0.2	0.03	0.27	1.8
1 tablespoon brewers' yeast	4	11	0.3	2.25	1.00	6.4
1 tablespoon blackstrap molasses	1	259	9.6	0.05	0.06	6.1
1 tablespoon white syrup	0	2	0	0	0	0

flour, 3 tablespoons wheat germ, 3 tablespoons soya flour, 4 tablespoons powdered skim milk, 2 teaspoons brown sugar, 1½ teaspoons vegetable salt (iodized). Dissolve ½ cake of yeast (½ ounce) in cup of lukewarm water (or leftover vegetable water) and add to dry ingredients. Also add 1 tablespoon margarine and mix thoroughly. Put the smooth dough in an oiled bowl and cover. Let rise in warm place for 1½ hours. Then punch down and let rise 20 minutes more. Finally make a loaf and put in large bread pan, cover, and let stand in warm place. When dough has again risen to top of bread pan, bake for about 40 minutes at 400 degrees F.

Whole Wheat Rolls

Mix ½ cup scalded fortified milk, 2 tablespoons butter, 1 tablespoon honey, and 1 teaspoon iodized vegetable salt. Cool this mixture to lukewarm temperature by adding ½ cup water (or leftover vegetable water). Add 1 cake compressed yeast, blend in 1 beaten egg, and finally add 3 cups whole wheat flour and 2 tablespoons wheat germ. Let rise in warm place until the bulk is doubled. Form in rolls and place in buttered muffin pan. Bake at 400 degrees F. for just 20 minutes.

I dedicate this recipe to Rose Parker of Detroit, Michigan, who first fed me these delicious rolls.

Quick Whole Wheat Bread

Make same mixture as for whole wheat rolls; knead and place in bread tin. Bake at 375 degrees F. for 1 hour. Makes one delicious loaf.

Four-Star Soya Muffins

Take 1½ cups soya flour, 2 teaspoons baking powder, 1½ teaspoons iodized vegetable salt, 2 fresh eggs, 3 tablespoons brown sugar, 1 tablespoon grated orange rind, 1 cup fortified milk, 1 tablespoon melted butter, ¼ cup floured raisins, and ¼ cup floured walnut meats. Sift together the flour, baking powder, and salt. Separate the eggs and beat the yolks until very light and frothy. Beat the sugar into the egg yolks, add the orange rind, milk, and butter, and mix well. Pour the egg mixture into the dry ingredients and mix. Add the raisins and nut meats and mix thoroughly. Fold in the egg whites beaten stiff. Pour into small muffin tins and bake in slow oven, 300 degrees F., for about 35 minutes.

These are Paulette Goddard's favorite muffins and I dedicate this recipe to her.

Sunday Breakfast Puffs

Break 1 compressed yeast cake into ¼ cup lukewarm water. Scald 1 cup milk and add 1 teaspoon vegetable salt, 2 tablespoons brown sugar, and ½ cup margarine. Let cool until lukewarm, and add the yeast. Now stir in 2 well-beaten eggs, add 3 cups whole wheat flour (sifted), 2 tablespoons wheat germ, and 2 tablespoons soya flour, and mix well. Set bowl in warm place and let rise for 1½ to 2 hours. Then drop by spoonfuls into oiled muffin pans, filling cups only half full. Make a mixture of ¼ cup brown sugar, ½ teaspoon cinnamon, and ¼ cup chopped nuts, and sprinkle on top of each muffin. Let rise again until double in bulk, and bake in moderate oven (375 degrees F.) for 25 minutes. Delicious for Sunday brunch.

Wheat Germ Muffins

Mix 1 tablespoon honey and 1 tablespoon margarine. Combine ½ cup wheat germ, ¼ cup sifted whole wheat flour, ¼ cup sifted soya flour, ½ teaspoon baking soda, a pinch of vegetable salt. Add honey mixture to dry ingredients alternately with ¾ cup yogurt. Beat all thoroughly. Put into muffin tins and bake for 35 minutes at 350 degrees F. Very delicious and nourishing.

Reducing Muffins

Beat 1 fresh egg and add ½ cup leftover vegetable water. Sift ¾ cup gluten flour and ¼ teaspoon baking powder together, and add to vegetable water. Beat until smooth. Pour mixture into oiled muffin tin and bake in hot oven (400 degrees F.) for 15 minutes.

Soya Wheat Muffins

Mix 1 tablespoon molasses and honey with 1 tablespoon melted margarine. Combine ¼ cup sifted whole wheat flour, ¼ cup wheat germ, ½ cup sifted soya flour, ½ teaspoon baking soda, a pinch of vegetable salt, and add alternately with ¾ cup yogurt to the sweet mixture. Beat very well, pour into oiled muffin tins, and bake in moderate oven (350 degrees F.) for 30 minutes.

Vienna Pie Crust

The best and easiest pie shells to make: simply mix 1 cup whole wheat flour, 1 tablespoon wheat germ, 1 tablespoon brown sugar, ½ teaspoon vegetable salt, and ¼ lb. of butter or margarine, with fork or pastry blender. When well mixed, turn into pie tin and press firmly against bottom and sides (no rolling necessary). Bake in medium oven (350 degrees F.) until golden brown. Makes 1 large or 6 individual pie shells. Excellent with fresh or honeyed fruits.

This recipe I dedicate to my sister-in-law, Mrs. Otto Robert Hauser of Milwaukee, who created this delicious dessert for me.

Delicious Waffles

Put 1 cake of yeast into 2 cups of warm yogurt or sour milk. To this add 3 egg yolks, 1 cup fresh wheat germ, 1 teaspoon vegetable salt, 1/3 cup butter, 1 tablespoon molasses and honey. Into these ingredients sift 1/3 cup dried skim milk and 1¼ cups whole wheat flour. Mix well, then place near stove or radiator and let rise for 1 to 2 hours. When bulk has doubled, stir with spoon. When ready to cook waffles, mix in 3 egg whites stiffly beaten. Serve hot, with molasses and honey or Five-minute Applesauce. This recipe I dedicate to Virginia Fox Kennady of Detroit, Michigan, an expert on both food and beauty.

Gayelord Hauser Cereal

For the best tasting and most nutritious cooked cereal, mix the following: 1 cup cracked whole wheat, ½ cup cracked rye,

¼ cup rice bran, 1 tablespoon each of soya flour, brewers' yeast, bone meal, and millet. Mix and keep in glass jar. Cook 1 cup of this mixture in 3 cups of boiling water for only 3 minutes.

Swiss Breakfast

Soak overnight 1 tablespoon Gayelord Hauser meal in 2 tablespoons water. Next morning, add juice of ½ lemon, 1 tablespoon condensed milk, and mix. Shred 1 large or 2 small unpeeled apples into cereal mixture, and sprinkle with 1 tablespoon each of wheat germ and honey. Serve at once.

This famous combination is the *muesli* served for breakfast and dinner at the Bircher-Benner sanatorium in Zurich. It can be further fortified with a tablespoon of powdered milk or a handful of walnuts. Instead of apples, also try peaches, berries, bananas, or any fruit in season.

Thermos Cooked Breakfast

Stir ½ cup Gayelord Hauser meal into 2 cups salted boiling water. Stir for 3 minutes and pour into wide-mouthed thermos bottle. Cork the bottle and lay it on its side, so cereal will be well done. Next morning you have a steaming hot cereal, ready to eat with honey and fortified milk. Cook all cereals in this easy way.

RICE, POTATOES, GREEN BEANS ALMANDINE
Indian Rice Casserole

Put in big bowl 2½ cups cooked brown rice, 2 eggs slightly beaten, 2 cups fortified warm milk, 2 cups finely chopped parsley, 1 cup grated American cheese, 2 tablespoons finely chopped onion, 1 teaspoon vegetable salt. Mix lightly to prevent mashing the cooked rice. Place in buttered casserole and bake in moderate oven (325 degrees F.) for 1 hour.

Wild Rice Hamburgers

Mix 2 cups cooked wild rice, ½ cup chopped hazel nuts or walnuts, and 1 slightly beaten egg. When well mixed, shape into patties, using 1 heaping tablespoonful for each, and fry in butter or peanut oil.

I served these patties, and broiled grapefruit, to Greta Garbo the first time she ate at my house. I dedicate this recipe to her.

Fortified Potatoes

It is much better to eat potatoes in place of foodless spaghetti, white rice, or noodles. One single potato contains as much vitamin C as a small glass of fruit juice, some iron, and many other minerals. To prevent the loss of these important nutrients, potatoes should be cooked or baked as quickly as possible. Scrub potatoes and bake until mealy. Cut in two, fortify each half with a bit of butter, parsley, chives, or caraway seeds.

Mashed Potatoes

Cook potatoes in jackets. Remove thin peeling, add handful of chopped parsley, 1 tablespoon of powdered milk, pinch of vegetable salt, and fresh milk. Whip until smooth and serve hot.

Potatoes for Reducers

Scrub large potatoes, do not peel. Cut in half and scoop out most of the middle portion, until only about ½ inch of potato is left lining the skin. Rub with oil and bake in very hot oven until brown and crispy. Delicious and satisfying.

Royal Hashed Potatoes

Melt 1 heaping tablespoon butter in heavy iron skillet. Add 2 cups unpeeled new potatoes, boiled and diced, and ¼ cup minced onion. Season with vegetable salt. Then add 3 tablespoons fortified milk and let cook without stirring until browned on the bottom. Fold over like an omelet, and serve garnished with parsley.

These are the favorite potatoes of Queen Alexandra of Yugoslavia. We ate them daily during their majesties' stay in America. I respectfully dedicate this recipe to her.

Green Beans Almandine

Short-cook the youngest and smallest green beans obtainable. Then sauté in golden brown butter. In another iron skillet have coarsely chopped dark-brown roasted almonds. Sprinkle the hot almonds over the very hot beans and serve at once. Any meal becomes a banquet with such a festive vegetable. I first ate Green Beans Almandine at the Bel-Air home of that famous hostess, Marian Mill Preminger, and dedicate this recipe to her.

For a complete lesson in short-cooking all vegetables, see *The Gayelord Hauser Cook Book.*

FORTIFY YOUR SALAD OIL

It is hard to believe, but in all America there is no 100% natural oil. It is all refined and purified, much the same as white flour, and much of the food value is lost, especially the fatty acids that are so necessary to health and good looks. Many skin problems are due to the use of these overly refined fats, especially the solidified or hydrogenated ones. Until some Southerner with foresight makes a natural peanut oil with all the fatty acids, or some Californian presses out an olive oil and does not denature it, I recommend that you buy the best brand of peanut or olive oil and fortify it with fresh wheat germ oil. Be sure it is the kind that has been extracted by the solvent process. You simply put a quart of peanut oil into a quart Mason jar and add 2 ounces of wheat germ oil. If you like the flavor of olive oil, add a handful of crushed ripe olives to this mixture, and you have one of the tastiest and certainly one of the most wholesome oils for your salads and for all cooking purposes. Remember that, with the exception of butter, vegetable fats are better for older people than animal fats. Liquid vegetable oils are better than the hardened or hydrogenated vegetable fats.

Peanut Oil Salad Dressing

Place in a pint Mason jar ¾ cup peanut oil, ¼ cup lemon juice or cider vinegar, 1 teaspoon iodized vegetable salt, 1 teaspoon brown sugar or honey, a dash each of garlic powder and mild paprika. Shake well before using, and keep cool in refrigerator.

Cream Cheese Dressing

Mix 4 tablespoons peanut oil, 2 tablespoons lemon juice, ½ teaspoon iodized vegetable salt, ½ teaspoon honey, and a dash of onion powder. Work this mixture into a 3-ounce package of cream cheese until soft and smooth. Delicious with raw vegetables in place of mayonnaise.

Florida Dressing

Mash very ripe avocados, or put in electric mixer. When smooth, use 1 cup avocado pulp and mix in ¼ cup lemon juice,

1 teaspoon iodized vegetable salt, 1 teaspoon brown sugar or honey, and, if you like, a dash of garlic. Blend well and serve with fruit salads.

Yogurt Mayonnaise

Mix 4 tablespoons fortified yogurt with 4 tablespoons peanut oil mayonnaise. Beat to consistency of thick cream. A tablespoon of finely chopped carrots or parsley makes this a delicious dressing for all vegetable combination salads.

Yogurt Salad Dressing for Reducers

Mix ½ teaspoon lemon juice or cider vinegar, ¼ teaspoon honey, a pinch of iodized vegetable salt, and the grated rind of ¼ lemon, into ½ cup fortified yogurt. To prevent monotony, vary the flavor by adding a bit of chives, watercress, or parsley. Delicious during elimination or reducing diets.

No-Oil Dressing

Make ½ cup of finely chopped young vegetables, as parsley, green onion, green pepper, radishes; mix with the liquid which has been pressed from a can of okra. Thin out with tomato juice. Season with iodized vegetable salt and a little honey. This is a delicious nonfattening salad dressing.

THE FAMILY SALAD BOWL

More and more American families are getting the salad bowl habit. It's practical, it's time-saving; the salads are delicious and contain important nutrients. Before mealtime, the chilled green lettuce leaves are broken into smaller pieces and put into a large wooden bowl which has been lightly rubbed with garlic. Add any other ingredients your family likes—thin unpeeled cucumber slices, tomatoes, radishes, green peppers, watercress—the more variety the better. Put the bowl on the table, and when everyone is seated, pour over the salad your fortified oil, add some vegetable salt, a pinch of sugar, and last, some lemon juice or wine vinegar, and toss with a wooden fork and spoon. Now add 1 or 2 tablespoons fresh wheat germ and toss some more. Serve at once at the beginning of meal, and watch this salad treat disappear.

For 100 different salad combinations, I suggest you study *The Gayelord Hauser Cook Book*.

Finger Salad

Most people like to munch fresh crisp vegetables in the "raw." It is no longer chic, and certainly not wise, to serve overrich, fat-laden appetizers which spoil the appetite for a good dinner. Why not serve finger salad at your next cocktail party? Also, if your waistline is out of bounds, why not get the habit and learn to enjoy the natural flavor of vegetables. Fix a tray with the following: Tender carrot sticks; bits of raw cauliflower; slices of green and red peppers (every Hungarian's delight); red and white radishes; young onions; celery and *fenucchi* sticks; whole small tomatoes. Have a shaker of vegetable salt handy for extra flavor and, if some guests insist on a dressing, have a bowl of chilled yogurt dressing and let them dip their vegetables into this refreshing and not greasy dressing.

DESSERTS IN THE MODERN MANNER
Yogurt Pie

The pride and joy of the Farmer's Market in Hollywood is yogurt pie. Everyone exclaims over it, and at the elaborate parties of the stars, this is the favorite dessert. You simply fill an 8-inch pastry shell with the following: 1 cup thick fortified yogurt, ½ pound mild cream cheese, 1 tablespoon honey, and ½ teaspoon vanilla. All are whipped together to the consistency of heavy whipped cream, poured into the pastry shell, and placed in refrigerator until served. Or you can make individual yogurt pies, filling the bottom with honeyed strawberries or pineapple, and placing the yogurt mixture on top.

I dedicate this delicious recipe to vivacious Cobina Wright Sr., my neighbor in Beverly Hills, California, who first discovered yogurt pie at the Farmer's Market and raved about it in her column.

Delicious Pound Cake

Cream 1 pound of butter. Gradually add 2 cups brown sugar and pinch of salt, and cream together until fluffy. Add 6 egg yolks one at a time, and beat well. Add 2 cups sifted whole wheat flour, grated rind of 2 large oranges, and juice of 1 orange. Beat egg whites stiff and fold into mixture. Bake in loaf pan at 300 degrees F. for 1 hour.

Fortified Custard

To your favorite custard recipe, simply add 2 heaping tablespoons powdered skim milk mixed into the sweet milk, and use natural dark brown sugar in place of white sugar.

Yogurt Sherbet

Mix together ½ cup of your favorite fruit juice, ¼ cup honey; add to this 1 cup fortified yogurt, 1 tablespoon lemon juice, a pinch of vegetable salt, and mix thoroughly. Transfer to freezing tray and freeze until firm. Then remove into bowl and stir well until free from lumps. Now add 2 egg whites, beaten stiff, folding into the smooth mixture. Return to freezing tray. A variety of fortified sherbets can be made with crushed pineapple, grape juice, fresh orange juice.

Honeyed Rice Pudding

Wash 3 tablespoons natural brown rice, and spread on bottom of buttered casserole. Mix 1 quart fortified milk (fortified skim milk, if this is for overweight diners), 2 tablespoons honey, and ½ teaspoon vegetable salt, and pour over rice. Now sprinkle in 2 tablespoons seedless raisins. Bake in moderate oven for 1½ hours. Chopped apricots or dates may be used in place of raisins.

Golden Apricot Soufflé

Soak ½ to ¾ pounds dried apricots (enough to make ¾ cup apricot purée) in warm water overnight. Press through sieve or put in mixer and purée. Beat 5 egg whites until stiff, and beat into them 5 tablespoons brown sugar and a pinch of vegetable salt. Fold into the apricot purée, pile lightly into a buttered baking dish, and bake in slow oven (300 degrees F.) until center is firm, about 45 minutes. Served with vanilla or fruit sauce, it makes a festive dessert. I dedicate this recipe to Princesse Windish-Graetz, one of America's great hostesses.

Honeyed Dried Fruit

Wash prunes, apricots, or raisins; cover with warm water and 1 or 2 tablespoons orange blossom honey. Do not cook, but let soak 24 hours. Unbelievably delicious for breakfast, or as a dessert.

Fruit Compote à la Lady Mendl

Make a moderately sweet syrup with sugar and water, or honey and water. While it is cooking, pick over your favorite fresh fruit: berries, cherries, halved apricots, pears, etc. Pour the hot, hot syrup over the fruit. Cover immediately to prevent the delicate aroma from escaping, and when cool, put covered fruit in refrigerator until served.

I have seen princes and statesmen devour this delicious compote. I dedicate this recipe to Lady Mendl's chef, Monsieur Fraise, who first served it to me.

Broiled Grapefruit

Cut large juicy grapefruit in half. Cut sections, but not center. Place 1 teaspoon molasses and honey, plus ½ teaspoon butter, in center. Broil for ½ hour, with a little water in pan to prevent burning.

Five-Minute Applesauce

Melt some fresh butter in a heavy skillet. When the butter is hot and still golden, put in finely shredded apples, heat thoroughly, and turn over so the melted butter is mixed with all the apples. Just before serving, sprinkle with California honey, and for special occasions, sprinkle with toasted chopped almonds. Serve hot, directly from skillet.

I served this elegant dessert at the Main Chance Beauty Farm, and dedicate this recipe to Elizabeth Arden.

Prune Whip

Mix 1½ cups pitted and chopped prunes with ¼ cup molasses and honey, 1 tablespoon lemon juice, ½ teaspoon lemon rind and a pinch of vegetable salt. Fold in 2 egg whites, beaten stiff.

Apricot Whip

1½ cups of slightly cooked dried apricots are folded into 1 cup chilled yogurt, and sprinkled with honey and grated orange peel. Both prune and apricot whip make delicious fillings for Continental pie shells.

Molasses Meringue

Beat 2 egg whites until foamy. Then beat 1/3 cup molasses into the egg white until it stands up in peaks. Pile gently on top of pie, and place under broiler until brown.

MODERN BEVERAGES

When coffee is made in the modern manner, and taken in moderation, it cannot be harmful to healthy people. The best and least harmful method of making coffee is to extract the flavor but not the acids. Percolating is the least desirable method; it extracts all the acids. Drip or filtered coffee is more desirable. But best of all is coffee made with freshly boiled, extremely hot water, such as the glass vacuum coffee-makers make. Another favorite method is to put freshly ground coffee into a heated porcelain pot and pour scalding hot water over it. Let the coffee stand for exactly 5 minutes by the clock, then drain, and you have the delicious flavor without the bitter and harmful acids. If coffee does not agree with you, or if your doctor does not approve it, there are other delicious beverages to choose from.

Peppermint Tea

Put 1 teaspoonful of fragrant dried leaves to each cup of boiling water in the pot. Let simmer for 3 minutes, to extract the beneficial oils. Serve with lemon and honey. An excellent digestive.

Papaya Tea

Prepare the same as peppermint tea. Serve piping hot. Wonderful for oldsters with gas and digestive difficulties. May also be mixed with peppermint, or wild strawberry leaves. Tastes more like real tea but contains no harmful acids.

Hauser Cup

Put 1 tablespoon dry skim milk into a large cup. Fill cup with scalding hot water and stir with fork. When all milk is dissolved, add a pinch of vegetable salt and 2 teaspoons of blackstrap molasses and, if you like, a bit of fresh milk.

New Orleans Cup

Beat 2 teaspoons blackstrap molasses into a cup of scalding hot water; add a pinch of vegetable salt and flavor with fresh milk.

Good Night Cap

Beat 2 teaspoons blackstrap molasses into a cup of very hot milk. Get into bed, sip slowly, and pleasant dreams!

I dedicate and commend the above hot drinks to all those men and women who cannot drink coffee. Try them; they are delicious and let you sleep deeply and soundly.

SPECIAL PURPOSE RECIPES

Delicious Fruit Laxative

To make a delicious and effective fruit laxative, grind up 1 cup stoned dried prunes, 1 cup seedless raisins, 1 cup black California figs, and 3 teaspoons Swiss Kriss, the laxative herbs. Mix fruits and herbs in a bowl and put through food grinder. To prevent sticking, pour boiling hot water through grinder. Form mixture into balls the size of a small walnut, roll in brown sugar, and place in refrigerator. The most natural and effective laxative for older people.

Vitamin P Extract

Slice 3 unpeeled lemons, 1 unpeeled orange, and put into 1 quart water. Boil slowly for 10 minutes. Add 2 tablespoons honey and boil 5 minutes more. Drain off liquid and cool. Drink 3 glasses a day.

Vitamin P Marmalade

Use the thin peelings of 2 golden oranges, 2 lemons, ½ grapefruit. Chop all very fine and mix with 1 cup orange blossom honey.

How To Extract Vitamin C

During the war, vitamin C was extracted from green walnuts and pine needles. But the best and richest extract of Vitamin C can be obtained from rose hips. Simply put rose hips into boiling water and let simmer for 15 minutes, being sure to keep pot covered. Let stand overnight. Next morning, strain, add 2 tablespoons lemon juice to each pint, and keep in jars. Fortify all fruit or vegetable drinks with a tablespoon of this rich vitamin C extract.

Wheat Germ Candy

Place 1/3 cup molasses and honey in mixing bowl; gradually work into it 2/3 cup powdered skim milk, 1/3 cup fresh wheat germ. Knead mixture on board or table with more powdered milk if necessary. Form into pieces the size of a walnut, roll in brown sugar. A most nourishing and delicious candy.

Molasses Candy

Place the following ingredients in mixing bowl: ½ cup molasses and honey, ½ cup thick peanut butter, 1 cup powdered skim milk, ½ cup seedless raisins. Mix well, and knead on board with more powdered milk until stiff. Cut into small pieces and roll in brown sugar.

Reducing Candy

Mix 2 pounds 3 ounces dextrose, 8 ounces molasses and honey, 2 ounces butter, into 1 pint (16 ounces) water. Cook whole mixture, stirring vigorously and constantly, until temperature reaches 278 degrees F. as measured by thermometer. Then flavor with 1 teaspoon vanilla and pour mixture onto cold slab or enamel table. When cooled, work as you would taffy. The finished mixture is then rolled and cut into pieces the size of sugar cubes. Taking one of these candies, every hour on the hour, between meals, helps to prevent hunger pains and trains an unruly appetite.

Toasted Soya Nuts

Cover ½ cup dried soybeans with 1½ cups water and soak overnight. Next morning, put soaked beans into a towel and dry thoroughly. Put beans in heated heavy skillet and stir until beans are golden brown. Just before removing from skillet, add 1 tablespoon butter or peanut oil, and sprinkle with ½ teaspoon vegetable salt. A great success when served hot.

Soya Grits

Prepare soybeans as above; roast without fat or salt. When thoroughly roasted, let cool and put through food grinder or electric gadget. This makes an excellent breakfast cereal, or a substitute for expensive nut meats when sprinkled over cakes or cookies.

Garlic: A Friend in Disguise

Whether you love or hate garlic, the fact remains: it is a very wonderful plant. Both onions and garlic contain one of nature's potent germicides called acrolein. After onions or garlic are eaten, the mouth becomes clean and sterile, and halitosis is banished. Digestive disturbances, as gas and colitis, are unknown among the Slavic people who eat quantities of fresh and dried garlic. Some European doctors even insist that garlic, through its germicidal power, lowers high blood pressure. But more than any plant, garlic can give ordinary dishes character and distinction. Use it sparingly, though; a "suspicion" or *soupçon* only, as the French say. Some garlic fans like to take it in capsule form, but surely natural fresh garlic is much better. The next time your "inner man" is out of order, make this cream of garlic soup: Cut up 4 cloves of fresh garlic and cook for 5 minutes in a cup of fortified milk. Add a dash of vegetable salt, remove the cloves of garlic, and drink piping hot. Some garlic enthusiasts claim that this is the best sleep inducer. If you do not have fresh garlic, use ¼ teaspoon pure garlic powder, and let simmer for 5 minutes.

Super Tuber for Reducers

The Jerusalem artichoke, with its low starch content, is a boon to reducers and weight-watchers. It is called the Jerusalem artichoke because the Italians refer to it as "girasole" (artichoke of the sunflower). The tuber is actually a native of America. It is sometimes called Jerusalem potato but it has little resemblance to the "spud." The flavor of this vegetable is delicious and nutty, and has only 30 calories instead of 130, as the common potato. In Hollywood, at the Farmer's Market, these tubers are extremely popular. They can be baked and boiled and even make a good "mock potato" salad. By all means ask for this super tuber at your super market.

MY SEVEN DAY ELIMINATION DIET

CREATED THIS, which is probably my best-known diet, in 1922, when I started my first food clinic in Chicago. This was one of the most interesting periods in my long career. People came to me from all over the country—rich and poor, fat and thin, young and old. They were sick. They had "been everywhere, tried everything." Now they came to me as a last resort. Many were skeptical about trying "food science," as I then called it. I had to work fast to convince them, do something basic to help all these overfed and undernourished people—overfed with foodless starches and sugars, undernourished in proteins, vitamins, and minerals.

Like all overfed and undernourished people, they were saturated with waste and debris. Their bodies had become clogged and distended. Such clogging shows in many ways: as excess fat in obesity, as excess sugar in diabetes, as excess purine in rheumatism, and many other diseases of the blood vessels, the heart, the digestive apparatus. Even the brain and nerves can become overburdened with the body's auto-poisons. Over and over I explained to these people that uneliminated body wastes are the cause of many body difficulties, that body tissues must be constantly washed and cleansed or they become poisoned by their own wastes, that life and health depend upon the removal of the body's auto-poisons.

My Seven Day Elimination Diet is a Seven Day Housecleaning designed to help Nature in ridding the body of accumulated and unwanted food and waste residue. What it does is to saturate the body with optimum amounts of vitamins and minerals, give the "inner man" a much-needed rest from past dietetic mistakes, and give Nature a perfect opportunity to exert her marvelous capacity to reinforce the body.

You can go on this Seven Day Elimination Diet (actually it is a feast) whenever you feel the need for a thorough cleansing. Springtime is ideal, for the first vegetables and fruits coming from the garden are especially rich in vitamins and minerals. But here in America, where we have fresh fruits and vegetables the year around, the diet can be taken at any time of year. I, myself, and thousands of my students, go on the Seven Day Elimination Diet twice a year: before Easter to ward off allergies and "spring fever," and again in the fall to prevent the ills of winter. I am convinced that such periodic cleansings and removal of body wastes can prevent much suffering and premature aging.

Here, then, are the foods which you can eat to your heart's content for seven days and at the same time give your body a Seven Day Housecleaning:

BIRD'S-EYE VIEW OF THE SEVEN DAY ELIMINATION DIET

BREAKFAST: Upon arising, after cleansing your mouth, drink a large glass of fruit juice, preferably fresh, such as orange, grapefruit, pineapple, or apple juice. In addition to the fruit juice, you may have one or two cups of fragrant herb tea such as peppermint, strawberry, or papaya tea. These can be flavored with a bit of honey and a slice of lemon. It is best to do without coffee. However, if you simply cannot get along without it, have one cup of fresh coffee and drink it clear. Should the fruit juice and a hot beverage not satisfy you, you might add some fresh or stewed fruit sweetened with a little honey.

DURING THE MORNING: If you want something more substantial, have a cup of yogurt, plain or flavored. You could also have a "finger salad" consisting of celery sticks, carrot sticks, slice of green pepper or bits of cauliflower flavored with vegetable salt. If chewing is a problem, have a glass of vegetable juice.

LUNCHEON: One cup of hot broth, a fresh fruit or vegetable salad, a dish of yogurt, hot tea with lemon.

DURING THE AFTERNOON: A glass of your favorite fruit or vegetable juice, fresh if possible. If something hot is wanted, one cup of peppermint tea with lemon and honey.

DINNER: A cup of broth, one cooked vegetable, a fresh green salad, a cup of herb tea or demitasse.

BEDTIME: Take a 20-minute warm relaxing bath. If bowels do not move freely, take some mild herbal laxative. If hungry, have some fresh fruit, fruit juice, or fat-free yogurt.

You can make up your own menus from the list of fruits and vegetables that follows, or you can follow the day-by-day plan given further on. *The pint of yogurt which I have added to the daily menu is of great help, but do not use more than a pint if you are overweight, and be sure to remove the cream from the milk.*

HERE ARE THE FRUITS TO CHOOSE FROM

1st Choice: Oranges, grapefruit, pineapple (whole or in juice form), lemon and lime juices in water.
2nd Choice: Apples, peaches, grapes, pears, apricots, and all berries.
3rd Choice: All melons, also papayas, pomegranates, and persimmons. (No bananas during this week.)

HERE ARE THE VEGETABLES TO CHOOSE FROM

1st Choice: Celery, carrots, spinach, parsley, beet tops, watercress, and okra.
2nd Choice: Celery roots, cucumbers, asparagus, green and red peppers, bean sprouts, and eggplant.

3rd Choice: Red and white cabbage, sauerkraut, cauliflower, beets, zucchini, and young peas.

Cooked vegetables can be seasoned with soy sauce, not butter.

Don't let yourself get hungry. If you are working, take some fresh fruit, some celery and carrots to the office, so that you will have something to eat during the morning and afternoon.

First Day

BREAKFAST:	Large glass orange juice or grapefruit juice
	Hot beverage: your choice of: peppermint, papaya, or strawberry tea with a bit of honey. Clear coffee, if you must.
	If still hungry, you may add some fruit, as melon, berries, peaches or apples; pears, fresh or baked.
MIDMORNING:	Your choice of any *one* of the following:
	Fresh fruit in season or fruit juice (no bananas)
	Raw vegetables in season or vegetable juice
	Sauerkraut juice or tomato and sauerkraut juice (equal amounts mixed—an excellent reducing cocktail)
	Yogurt or buttermilk (not more than three cups a day)
	If you prefer something hot, your choice of: hot Hauser Broth, hot tomato juice, hot herb tea (peppermint, papaya, strawberry), weak tea with lemon—sweetened only with a bit of honey or brown sugar. Clear coffee, if you must.

LUNCHTIME:
Hot Hauser Broth or tomato juice
Yogurt or buttermilk—one cup
Salad: cucumber, lettuce, green pepper (or your own combination), with yogurt dressing
Choice of hot beverage as above

MIDAFTERNOON: Same as midmorning

DINNERTIME:
Hot Hauser Broth
Spinach, or other greens, steamed with thin slices of onion
Salad: sliced tomatoes
Yogurt or buttermilk
Baked apple
Choice of hot beverage as above

BEDTIME: Same as midmorning

Check up on your elimination. Take a simple herbal laxative when needed.

Second Day

BREAKFAST:
Large glass orange or grapefruit juice
Hot beverage: your choice of: peppermint, papaya, or strawberry tea with a bit of honey. Clear coffee, if you must.
If still hungry, you may add some fruit as melon, berries, peaches or apples; pears, fresh or baked.

MIDMORNING:
Your choice of any *one* of the following:
Fresh fruit in season (no bananas) or fruit juice
Raw vegetables in season or vegetable juice
Sauerkraut juice or tomato and sauerkraut juice (equal amounts mixed—an excellent reducing cocktail)

Yogurt or buttermilk (not more than three cups a day)

If you prefer something hot, your choice of: one or two cups hot Hauser Broth, hot tomato juice, hot herb tea (peppermint, papaya, strawberry), weak tea with lemon —sweetened only with a bit of honey or brown sugar. Clear coffee, if you must.

LUNCHTIME: Hot Hauser Broth or tomato juice
                    Yogurt or buttermilk—one cup
                    Salad: pineapple, carrot, and raisins
                    Choice of hot beverage as above

MIDAFTERNOON: Same as midmorning

DINNERTIME: Hot Hauser Broth
                    Steamed cauliflower
                    Salad: celery hearts and strips of green peppers
                    Yogurt or buttermilk
                    Fresh or broiled grapefruit
                    Choice of hot beverage as above

BEDTIME: Same as midmorning.

Check up on your elimination. Take a simple herbal laxative when needed.

Third Day

BREAKFAST: Large glass orange or grapefruit juice
                    Hot beverage: your choice of: peppermint, papaya, or strawberry tea with a bit of honey. Clear coffee, if you must.
                    If still hungry, you may add some fruit as melon, berries, peaches or apples; pears, fresh or baked.

MIDMORNING:	Your choice of any *one* of the following:
	Fresh fruit in season (no bananas) or fruit juice
	Raw vegetables in season or vegetable juice
	Sauerkraut juice or tomato and sauerkraut juice (equal amounts mixed—an excellent reducing cocktail)
	Yogurt or buttermilk (not more than three cups a day)
	If you prefer something hot, your choice of: one or two cups hot Hauser Broth, hot tomato juice, hot herb tea (peppermint, papaya, strawberry), weak tea with lemon —sweetened only with a bit of honey or brown sugar. Clear coffee, if you must.
LUNCHTIME:	Hot Hauser Broth or tomato juice
	Salad: cabbage and pineapple with yogurt dressing
	Yogurt or buttermilk
	Choice of hot beverage as above
MIDAFTERNOON:	Same as midmorning
DINNERTIME:	Hot Hauser Broth
	Broiled eggplant (inch-thick slices) or summer squash
	Salad: sliced cucumbers
	Yogurt or buttermilk
	Fresh or stewed fruit
	Choice of hot beverage as above
BEDTIME:	Same as midmorning

Check up on your elimination, taking a simple herbal laxative when needed.

Fourth Day

BREAKFAST:
Large glass orange or grapefruit juice
Hot beverage: your choice of: peppermint, papaya, or strawberry tea with a bit of honey. Clear coffee, if you must.
If still hungry, you may add some fruit as melon, berries, peaches or apples; pears, fresh or baked

MIDMORNING:
Your choice of any *one* of the following:
Fresh fruit in season (no bananas), or fruit juice
Raw vegetables in season or vegetable juice
Sauerkraut juice or tomato and sauerkraut juice (equal amounts mixed—an excellent reducing cocktail)
Yogurt or buttermilk (not more than three cups a day)
If you prefer something hot, your choice of: one or two cups of hot Hauser Broth, hot tomato juice, hot herb tea (peppermint, papaya, strawberry), weak tea with lemon —sweetened only with a bit of honey or brown sugar. Clear coffee, if you must.

LUNCHTIME:
Hot Hauser Broth or tomato juice
Salad: apple, celery, and orange diced
Choice of hot beverage as above

MIDAFTERNOON: Same as midmorning

DINNERTIME:
Hot Hauser Broth
Stewed tomatoes
Finger salad: celery and carrot sticks and green onions
Yogurt or buttermilk

Berries or fruit in season
Choice of hot beverage as above

BEDTIME: Same as midmorning

Check up on your elimination. Take a simple herbal laxative when needed.

Fifth Day

BREAKFAST: Large glass orange or grapefruit juice
Hot beverage: your choice of: peppermint, papaya, or strawberry tea, with a bit of honey. Clear coffee, if you must.
If still hungry, you may add some fresh fruit as melon, berries, peaches or apples; pears, fresh or baked.

MIDMORNING: Your choice of any *one* of the following:
Fresh fruit in season or fruit juice (no bananas)
Raw vegetables in season or vegetable juice
Sauerkraut juice or tomato and sauerkraut juice (equal amounts mixed—an excellent reducing cocktail)
Yogurt or buttermilk (not more than three cups a day)
If you prefer something hot, your choice of: one or two cups hot Hauser Broth, hot tomato juice, hot herb tea (peppermint, papaya, strawberry), weak tea with lemon —sweetened only with a bit of honey or brown sugar. Clear coffee, if you must.

LUNCHTIME: Hot Hauser Broth or tomato juice
Yogurt or buttermilk
Salad: fruit salad
Choice of hot beverage as above

MIDAFTERNOON: Same as midmorning

DINNERTIME: Hot Hauser Broth
                Vegetable Chop Suey (equal amounts of
                    diced celery, onions, and bean sprouts
                    when available, seasoned with soy sauce)
                Salad: sliced tomatoes
                Yogurt or buttermilk
                Peaches or fruit in season
                Choice of hot beverage as above

BEDTIME: Same as midmorning

Check up on your elimination, taking a simple herbal laxative
when needed.

Sixth Day

BREAKFAST: Large glass orange or grapefruit juice
                Hot beverage: your choice of: peppermint,
                    papaya, or strawberry tea with a bit of
                    honey. Clear coffee, if you must.
                If still hungry, you may add some fruit as
                    melon, berries, peaches or apples; pears,
                    fresh or baked.

MIDMORNING: Your choice of any *one* of the following:
                Fresh fruit in season or fruit juice (no ba-
                    nanas)
                Raw vegetables in season or vegetable juice
                Sauerkraut juice or tomato and sauerkraut
                    juice (equal amounts mixed—an excellent
                    reducing cocktail)
                Yogurt or buttermilk (not more than three
                    cups a day)
                If you prefer something hot, your choice of:
                    one or two cups hot Hauser Broth, hot to-
                    mato juice, hot herb tea (peppermint,
                    papaya, strawberry), weak tea with lemon

—sweetened only with honey or brown
sugar. Clear coffee, if you must.

LUNCHTIME: Hot Hauser Broth or tomato juice
Yogurt or buttermilk
Finger salad: cauliflower buds, green onions,
carrot and celery sticks, and other raw
vegetables in season
Choice of hot beverage as above

MIDAFTERNOON: Same as midmorning

DINNERTIME: Hot Hauser Broth
Stew of tomatoes, onions, and green peppers
—okra if available
Salad: chopped pineapple, carrot, and cab-
bage
Yogurt or buttermilk
Fresh pears or fruit in season
Choice of hot beverage as above

BEDTIME: Same as midmorning

Check up on your elimination. Take a simple herbal laxative
when needed.

Seventh Day

BREAKFAST: Large glass orange or grapefruit juice
Hot beverage: your choice of: peppermint,
papaya, or strawberry tea with a bit of
honey. Clear coffee, if you must.
If still hungry, you may add some fresh fruit
as melon, berries, peaches or apples; pears,
fresh or baked.

MIDMORNING: Your choice of any *one* of the following:
Fresh fruit in season or fruit juice (no ba-
nanas)
Raw vegetables in season or vegetable juice
Sauerkraut juice or tomato and sauerkraut

juice (equal amounts mixed—an excellent reducing cocktail)

Yogurt or buttermilk (not more than three cups a day)

If you prefer something hot, your choice of: one or two cups hot Hauser Broth, hot tomato juice, hot herb tea (peppermint, papaya, strawberry), weak tea with lemon —sweetened only with honey or brown sugar. Clear coffee, if you must.

LUNCHTIME:

Hot Hauser Broth or tomato juice

Yogurt or buttermilk

Salad: raw sauerkraut with lemon juice

Choice of hot beverage as above

MIDAFTERNOON: Same as midmorning

DINNERTIME:

Hot Hauser Broth

Cooked young green peas

Salad: chopped celery hearts and watercress and orange

Yogurt or buttermilk—one cup

Sliced pineapple or fruit in season

Choice of hot beverage as above

BEDTIME: Same as midmorning

Check up on your elimination. Take a simple herbal laxative when needed.

Hauser Broth

1 cup finely shredded celery, leaves and all
1 cup finely shredded carrots
½ cup shredded spinach
1 tablespoon shredded parsley
1 teaspoon vegetable salt
1 quart water

    1 cup tomato juice
    Brown sugar or honey

Put all shredded vegetables into the quart of water, cover and cook slowly for about 25 minutes, then add tomato juice, a teaspoon vegetable salt, and a pinch of brown sugar or honey. Let cook for a few more minutes. Strain and serve.

Should you be hungry as a bear and *not* overweight, you may eat the broth unstrained. Added vegetable juices give variety and flavor to the broth. If you are unable to buy them and do not possess a juicer, you may add any of your favorite vegetables or herbs. Some days add a bit of onion (fresh or dried flakes), green peppers, beet tops, chives, etc. This broth has been a "comfort to thousands" as Billie Burke once wrote, and is the same formula I served on Elizabeth Arden's beauty farm. It has been used since by many of the other Fifth Avenue beauty studios. If you are unable to prepare this broth, you can use any prepared dry vegetable broth and heat it to simmering point in tomato juice. Or you can buy canned mixed vegetable juice, flavor it with vegetable salt, and heat, but do not boil.

LIVE LONGER REDUCING PLAN

HEN you have made up your mind that you really *want* to reduce, let these menus guide you until you have learned to enjoy low calorie foods. To help you train your turbulent and demanding stomach, make brewers' yeast, fortified skim milk, and lean proteins your main standbys. Acquire the excellent habit of putting a tablespoon of brewers' yeast in a glass of tomato or mixed vegetable juice, and drinking it before each meal. This helps to destroy the appetite for more fattening foods, gives extra proteins and B vitamins to prevent lines and wrinkles. Here is what you can look forward to each and every day:

BREAKFAST: One tablespoon of good-tasting powdered brewers' yeast mixed into a glass of tomato juice, grapefruit juice, or orange juice. If unable to take powdered brewers' yeast with breakfast, take 6 standardized yeast tablets containing the entire B family. PLUS one egg poached, boiled, or scrambled in milk, or three slices broiled lean bacon, or two tablespoons of chipped beef, or two tablespoons whole cereal. PLUS one thin slice of whole wheat toast or two rye crackers. PLUS glass of fortified milk or café au lait (equal amounts of coffee and hot milk). PLUS YOUR LIVE LONGER REDUCING RITUAL to prevent any possible shortage of important factors: 1 fish liver oil capsule for your vitamins A and D, 1 ascorbic acid tablet (100 milligrams) for your vitamin C, 1 wheat germ oil capsule (30 milligrams) for your vitamin E.

MIDMORNING: Your choice of: glass of celery juice, or fat-free yogurt, or large fresh tomato, or glass of fortified milk.

LUNCHEON: Glass of tomato juice with tablespoon of powdered brewers' yeast. PLUS generous helping of lean meat or fish or cottage cheese or fortified milk soup or omelet or baked soya beans. PLUS finger salad: carrot sticks, celery sticks, tomatoes, cucumber sticks, cauliflower, fenucchi, etc. PLUS glass of fat-free yogurt, flavored with cinnamon or nutmeg or one teaspoon blackstrap molasses. PLUS beverage: tea with lemon, or black coffee.

MIDAFTERNOON: Same as midmorning, or a glass of cold or hot tomato juice fortified with one tablespoon of powdered brewers' yeast.

DINNER: Your choice: clear bouillon or vegetable soup. PLUS generous helping of lean meat, fish, fowl, liver broiled or roasted.

PLUS one cooked leafy vegetable (little fat). PLUS salad of finely chopped raw vegetables, blended with fat-free yogurt or cottage cheese. PLUS beverage: café au lait or demitasse.

BEDTIME: Cold or hot fortified milk or yogurt, or hot tomato juice fortified with powdered brewers' yeast.

Here are some easy-to-follow REDUCING MENUS:

BREAKFAST:	Fortified grapefruit juice One poached egg Two rye crackers Glass of fortified milk or café au lait
	Your Live Longer Reducing Ritual: 1 fish liver oil capsule, 1 ascorbic acid tablet, 1 wheat germ oil capsule and, if your juice was not fortified, also take 6 standardized yeast tablets. Drink all down with your beverage.
MIDMORNING:	Glass of celery juice or fat-free yogurt or large fresh tomato or glass of fortified milk
LUNCHEON:	Fortified tomato juice Omelet baked in milk Finger salad Yogurt flavored with cinnamon Tea with lemon, or café au lait
MIDAFTERNOON:	Glass of fortified mixed vegetable or tomato juice
DINNER:	Large broiled hamburger String beans Tomato salad Fortified milk or demitasse
BEDTIME:	Hot or cold fortified milk

BREAKFAST:

Fortified orange juice
Three slices lean crisp bacon
Two rye crackers
Glass of fortified milk or café au lait

Your Live Longer Reducing Ritual: 1 fish liver oil capsule, 1 ascorbic acid tablet, 1 wheat germ oil capsule and, if your juice was not fortified, also take 6 standardized yeast tablets. Drink all down with your beverage.

MIDMORNING:

Glass of celery juice or fat-free yogurt or fresh tomato or glass of fortified milk

LUNCHEON:

Fortified tomato juice
Two hard-boiled eggs
Finger salad
Fat-free yogurt flavored with grated lemon peel
Tea with lemon or café au lait

MIDAFTERNOON:

Glass of fortified tomato juice or mixed vegetable juice

DINNER:

Jellied bouillon
Large green pepper stuffed with lean ground round steak
Steamed summer squash
Tomato gelatin salad with cottage cheese
Fortified milk or demitasse

BEDTIME:

Hot or cold fortified milk

BREAKFAST:

Fortified tomato juice
One boiled egg, cooked firm
Two rye crackers
Glass of fortified milk or café au lait

Your Live Longer Reducing Ritual: 1 fish liver oil capsule, 1 ascorbic acid tablet, 1 wheat germ oil capsule and, if your juice was not fortified, also take 6 standardized yeast tablets. Drink all down with your beverage.

MIDMORNING: Glass of celery juice or fat-free yogurt or large fresh tomato or glass of fortified milk

LUNCHEON: Fortified tomato juice
Large cottage cheese salad, yogurt dressing
Finger salad
Fat-free yogurt flavored with grated orange peel
Tea with lemon or café au lait

MIDAFTERNOON: Glass of fortified tomato or mixed vegetable juice

DINNER: Shrimp cocktail
Broiled calves' liver
Salad bowl
Fortified milk or demitasse

BEDTIME: Hot or cold fortified milk

BREAKFAST: Fortified grapefruit juice
Two tablespoons of cooked whole wheat cereal with fortified milk and level teaspoon of honey
Glass of fortified milk or café au lait

Your Live Longer Reducing Ritual: 1 fish liver oil capsule, 1 ascorbic acid tablet, 1 wheat germ oil capsule and, if your juice was not fortified, also take 6 standardized yeast tablets. Drink all down with your beverage.

MIDMORNING: Glass of celery juice or fat-free yogurt or
               large fresh tomato or glass of fortified milk

LUNCHEON: Fortified tomato juice
               Large slice of roast beef or leftover meats
               Finger salad
               Yogurt flavored with nutmeg
               Tea with lemon or café au lait

MIDAFTERNOON: Glass of fortified tomato or vegetable juice

DINNER: Hot broth
               Large helping lean fish
               Stewed tomatoes
               Cucumber salad
               Fortified milk or demitasse

BEDTIME: Hot or cold fortified milk

BREAKFAST: Fortified tomato juice
               Three slices lean crisp bacon
               One whole wheat muffin

               Your Live Longer Reducing Ritual: 1 fish
               liver oil capsule, 1 ascorbic acid tablet, 1
               wheat germ oil capsule and, if your juice
               was not fortified, also take 6 standardized
               yeast tablets. Drink all down with your
               beverage.

MIDMORNING: Glass of celery juice or fat-free yogurt or
               large fresh tomato or glass of fortified milk

LUNCHEON: Fortified vegetable juice
               Two hard-boiled eggs
               One cup coleslaw
               Fat-free yogurt
               Tea with lemon or café au lait

MIDAFTERNOON: Glass of fortified tomato or vegetable juice

DINNER:
 Large lean hamburger
 Cooked green vegetable
 Finger salad
 Fortified milk or demitasse

BEDTIME:
 Hot or cold fortified milk

BREAKFAST:
 Fortified grapefruit juice
 Swiss breakfast with nuts
 Glass of fortified milk or café au lait

 Your Live Longer Reducing Ritual: 1 fish liver oil capsule, 1 ascorbic acid tablet, 1 wheat germ oil capsule and, if your juice was not fortified, also take 6 standardized yeast tablets. Drink all down with your beverage.

MIDMORNING:
 Glass of celery juice or fat-free yogurt or large fresh tomato or glass of fortified milk

LUNCHEON:
 Fortified tomato juice
 Two broiled frankfurters
 Finger salad
 Fat-free yogurt
 Tea with lemon or café au lait

MIDAFTERNOON:
 Glass of fortified tomato or vegetable juice

DINNER:
 Half broiled chicken
 Cooked spinach or beet greens
 Gelatin salad with cottage cheese
 Fortified milk or demitasse

BEDTIME:
 Hot or cold fortified milk

BREAKFAST:
 Fortified orange juice
 One poached egg
 Two rye crackers
 Glass of fortified milk or café au lait

Your Live Longer Reducing Ritual: 1 fish liver oil capsule, 1 ascorbic acid tablet, 1 wheat germ oil capsule and, if your juice was not fortified, also take 6 standardized yeast tablets. Drink all down with your beverage.

MIDMORNING:
Glass of celery juice or fat-free yogurt or large fresh tomato or glass of fortified milk

LUNCHEON:
Fortified tomato juice
Large chicken salad
Finger salad
Fat-free yogurt
Tea with lemon or café au lait

MIDAFTERNOON:
Glass of fortified tomato or vegetable juice

DINNER:
Fresh vegetable juice
Broiled liver
Smothered onions and apples
Stewed pears
Fortified milk or demitasse

BEDTIME:
Hot or cold fortified milk

BREAKFAST:
Fortified tomato juice
One egg scrambled in milk
Two rye crackers
Glass of fortified milk or café au lait

Your Live Longer Reducing Ritual: 1 fish liver oil capsule, 1 ascorbic acid tablet, 1 wheat germ oil capsule and, if your juice was not fortified, also take 6 standardized yeast tablets. Drink all down with your beverage.

MIDMORNING:
Glass of celery juice or fat-free yogurt or large fresh tomato or glass of fortified milk

LUNCHEON: Fortified tomato juice
Two tablespoons chipped beef creamed with milk
Finger salad
Fat-free yogurt
Tea with lemon or café au lait

MIDAFTERNOON: Glass of fortified tomato or mixed vegetable juice

DINNER: Vegetable soup
Large helping of lean beef
Green or yellow beans
Fresh berries with yogurt
Fortified milk or demitasse

BEDTIME: Hot or cold fortified milk

BREAKFAST: Fortified grapefruit juice
Soya waffle
One teaspoon honey
Glass of fortified milk or café au lait

Your Live Longer Reducing Ritual: 1 fish liver oil capsule, 1 ascorbic acid tablet, 1 wheat germ oil capsule and, if your juice was not fortified, also take 6 standardized yeast tablets. Drink all down with your beverage.

MIDMORNING: Glass of celery juice or fat-free yogurt or large fresh tomato or glass of fortified milk

LUNCHEON: Fortified tomato juice
Four heaping teaspoons of cottage cheese on sliced tomatoes
Fat-free yogurt
Tea with lemon or café au lait

MIDAFTERNOON: Glass of fortified tomato or mixed vegetable juice

DINNER: Large helping pounded round steak
Stewed tomatoes and green peppers
Carrot and celery sticks
Fortified milk or demitasse

BEDTIME: Hot or cold fortified milk

BREAKFAST: Fortified tomato juice
Shredded wheat biscuits with berries and milk
Glass of fortified milk or café au lait

Your Live Longer Reducing Ritual: 1 fish liver oil capsule, 1 ascorbic acid tablet, 1 wheat germ oil capsule and, if your juice was not fortified, also take 6 standardized yeast tablets. Drink all down with your beverage.

MIDMORNING: Glass of celery juice or fat-free yogurt or large fresh tomato or glass of fortified milk

LUNCHEON: Two-egg Spanish omelet
Finger salad
Fat-free yogurt
Tea with lemon or demitasse

MIDAFTERNOON: Glass of fortified tomato or mixed vegetable juice

DINNER: Hot soup or salad bowl
Large portion of veal steak breaded with wheat germ
Cooked green vegetables
Fortified milk or demitasse

BEDTIME: Hot or cold fortified milk

Use these menus as a guide until you have learned to use more proteins, more vitamin-rich foods, and less starches, fats, and sugars. Break yourself of the five bad habits:

    the fancy dessert habit
    the bread with your meals habit
    the cream and sugar habit
    the cooking your vegetables to death habit
    the feeling sorry for yourself habit

and you will have solved your reducing problems for the rest of your long life. I highly recommend this diet to Eaters Anonymous and all those who have to lose 20 or more pounds. If you are only 10 pounds overweight and would like to lose it more quickly, I can recommend my very efficient and easy-to-follow POUND-A-DAY REDUCING DIET. Sometimes a new job, a new beau, or a new dress, may be the incentive. Contrary to popular opinion, there is no scientific evidence that more rapid reduction is harmful, especially if the reducing diet contains all the nutrients the body needs. The bad effects of haphazard diets have always been due to imbalance, or to harmful drugs. With this pound-a-day reducing diet, thousands of men and women have lost 10 pounds in 10 days. I recommend that this diet is followed for 10 days only. If more than 10 pounds need to be lost, the Live Longer Reducing Diet should be followed until the ideal weight (see chart on page 104) is reached.

THE POUND-A-DAY REDUCING DIET

This diet again uses plenty of protein foods, for they, more than any others, *satisfy*. Also, first class protein foods have a specific dynamic action and help to burn up fat. Since an all-protein diet could create too much acidity, the diet must also contain fruits, vegetables, and milk. The vitamins and minerals which are especially needed during the 10-day period are vitamins A, B, C, D, and E, plus the minerals calcium, phosphorus, iron, and iodine. These can largely be obtained from green and yellow vegetables and their juices, powdered brewers' yeast, and powdered skim milk, but so that there is no possibility of cheating the body, I recommend fortification with 1 fish liver oil capsule, 1 ascorbic acid tablet, 1 wheat germ capsule, and 4 mineral tablets containing calcium, phosphorus, iron, and the very important organic iodine, to be taken each and every day, preferably right at breakfast. Here are the menus which will help you to be 10 pounds lighter and much brighter in exactly 10 short days:

MENUS FOR TEN DAYS
First Day

BREAKFAST:

Half a grapefruit
Clear coffee or café au lait

Fortify yourself with 1 fish liver oil capsule, 1 ascorbic acid tablet, 1 wheat germ capsule, and your mineral tablets containing calcium, phosphorus, iron, and iodine.

LUNCH:

Two hard-boiled eggs topped with a half cup tomatoes
Fortified milk or clear beverage

DINNER:

Two lean hamburgers
Half a head of lettuce
Fresh or broiled grapefruit
Fortified milk or demitasse

BEDTIME:

Hot or cold fortified milk or glass of fortified tomato juice or glass of fat-free yogurt.
Check up on your vitamins and minerals.

If hungry between meals, eat celery, carrots, or a glass of fortified milk or tomato juice.

Second Day

BREAKFAST:
Half a grapefruit
Clear coffee

Fortify yourself with 1 fish liver oil capsule, 1
ascorbic acid tablet, 1 wheat germ capsule,
and your mineral tablets containing calcium, phosphorus, iron, and iodine.

LUNCH:
Four tablespoons of cottage cheese mixed
with chopped carrots
One slice rye bread toast
Fortified milk or clear beverage

DINNER:
Broiled half chicken
Half a cup spinach or beet greens
Mixed green salad
Baked apple

BEDTIME:
Hot or cold fortified milk or glass of fortified
tomato juice or glass of fat-free yogurt

If hungry between meals eat celery, carrots, or a glass of fortified
milk or tomato juice.

Third Day

BREAKFAST:
Half a grapefruit
Clear coffee

Fortify yourself with 1 fish liver oil capsule,
1 ascorbic acid tablet, 1 wheat germ capsule, and your mineral tablets containing
calcium, phosphorus, iron, and iodine.

LUNCH:
Two scrambled eggs
One slice rye bread toast
Large sliced tomato
Fortified milk or clear beverage

DINNER:
 Lean steak
 Salad bowl
 Fresh or broiled grapefruit
 Fortified milk or demitasse

BEDTIME:
 Hot or cold fortified milk or glass of fortified
 tomato juice or glass of fat-free yogurt

If hungry between meals, eat celery, carrots, or a glass of fortified milk or tomato juice.

Fourth Day

BREAKFAST:
 Half a grapefruit
 Clear coffee

 Fortify yourself with 1 fish liver oil capsule,
 1 ascorbic acid tablet, 1 wheat germ capsule, and your mineral tablets containing
 calcium, phosphorus, iron, and iodine.

LUNCH:
 Broiled round steak
 Watercress or lettuce salad
 One bran muffin
 Fortified milk or clear beverage

DINNER:
 Broiled lean fish
 Half a cup stewed tomatoes
 Coleslaw
 Baked apple
 Fortified milk or demitasse

BEDTIME:
 Hot or cold fortified milk or glass of fortified
 tomato juice or glass of fat-free yogurt

If hungry between meals, eat celery, carrots, or a glass of fortified milk or tomato juice.

Fifth Day

BREAKFAST:
Half a grapefruit
Clear coffee

Fortify yourself with 1 fish liver oil capsule,
1 ascorbic acid tablet, 1 wheat germ capsule and your mineral tablets containing
calcium, phosphorus, iron, and iodine.

LUNCH:
Two hard-boiled eggs topped with half a cup
spinach
Applesauce
Fortified milk or clear beverage

DINNER:
Broiled beef tenderloin or lean steak
Half a cup broccoli or cauliflower
Half a cup fruit salad
Fortified milk or demitasse

BEDTIME:
Hot or cold fortified milk or glass of fortified
tomato juice or glass of fat-free yogurt

If hungry between meals, eat celery, carrots, or a glass of fortified
milk or tomato juice.

Sixth Day

BREAKFAST:
Half a grapefruit
Clear coffee

Fortify yourself with 1 fish liver oil capsule, 1
ascorbic acid tablet, 1 wheat germ capsule,
and your mineral tablets containing calcium, phosphorus, iron, and iodine.

LUNCH:
One slice cheese on rye bread toast
Applesauce
Fortified milk or clear beverage

DINNER: · Two slices broiled liver
Half a cup cauliflower
Grapefruit salad
Fortified milk or demitasse

BEDTIME: Hot or cold fortified milk or glass of fortified
tomato juice or glass of fat-free yogurt

If hungry between meals, eat celery, carrots, or a glass of fortified milk or tomato juice.

Seventh Day (Sunday)

BREAKFAST: Half a grapefruit
Clear coffee

Fortify yourself with 1 fish liver oil capsule, 1
ascorbic acid tablet, 1 wheat germ capsule,
and your mineral tablets containing calcium, phosphorus, iron, and iodine.

LUNCH: Half a broiled chicken
Half a cup string beans
Half a cup fruit salad
Fortified milk or clear beverage

DINNER: Egg and celery salad (two chopped eggs with
chopped celery)
One slice rye bread toast
Fortified milk or demitasse

BEDTIME: Hot or cold fortified milk or glass of fortified
tomato juice or glass of fat-free yogurt

If hungry between meals, eat celery, carrots, or a glass of fortified milk or tomato juice.

Eighth Day

BREAKFAST:
Half a grapefruit
Clear coffee

Fortify yourself with 1 fish liver oil capsule, 1 ascorbic acid tablet, 1 wheat germ capsule, and your mineral tablets containing calcium, phosphorus, iron, and iodine.

LUNCH:
Large hamburger on rye bread toast
Sliced orange
Fortified milk or clear beverage

DINNER:
Two slices pot roast
Half a cup broccoli
Carrot sticks
Fresh or broiled grapefruit
Fortified milk or demitasse

BEDTIME:
Hot or cold fortified milk or glass of fortified tomato juice or glass of fat-free yogurt

If hungry between meals, eat celery, carrots or a glass of fortified milk or tomato juice.

Ninth Day

BREAKFAST:
Half a grapefruit
Clear coffee

Fortify yourself with 1 fish liver oil capsule, 1 ascorbic acid tablet, 1 wheat germ capsule, and your mineral tablets containing calcium, phosphorus, iron, and iodine.

LUNCH:
Waldorf salad with handful of nuts
One muffin
Fortified milk or clear beverage

DINNER: Lean fish
                        Stewed tomatoes
                        Cucumber and lettuce salad
                        Baked apple
                        Fortified milk or demitasse

BEDTIME: Hot or cold fortified milk or glass of fortified
                        tomato juice or glass of fat-free yogurt

If hungry between meals, eat celery, carrots, or a glass of fortified milk or tomato juice.

Tenth Day

BREAKFAST: Half a grapefruit
                        Clear coffee

                        Fortify yourself with 1 fish liver oil capsule, 1
                        ascorbic acid tablet, 1 wheat germ capsule,
                        and your mineral tablets containing cal-
                        cium, phosphorus, iron, and iodine.

LUNCH: Cold beef or lamb
                        Half a head lettuce
                        Applesauce
                        Fortified milk or clear beverage

DINNER: Mushroom omelet
                        Lettuce and tomato salad
                        Half a cup berries
                        Fortified milk or demitasse

BEDTIME: Hot or cold fortified milk or glass of fortified
                        tomato juice or glass of fat-free yogurt

If hungry between meals, eat celery, carrots, or a glass of fortified milk or tomato juice.

DON'T BE TOO THIN

*I*F YOU are slightly underweight, thank your lucky stars and stay that way. But if you are too thin, do something about it. Obviously you are not eating the right kind of food. Perhaps, also, you are too tense.

It is important that the diet eaten by thin people be rich in all body-building elements, especially the vitamins of the B family and the easily digested fatty acids found in vegetable oils, particularly peanut and wheat germ oils. If you are painfully thin and have not been able to gain in the past, by all means learn to "let go." Follow the relaxation exercise on page 338. The calcium foods and vitamin D are valuable in helping you to relax. These foods should be added to the daily diet in the form of fortified milk drinks, yogurt, cheese. If you are very tense and nervous, you can add some good calcium and vitamin D concentrate to your daily meals. Sunbaths are especially helpful to thin people because of their soothing and relaxing effect upon the whole body, plus the vitamin D direct sunshine imparts to the body. But do not overdo. See Dr. Rollier's technique (page 187).

While gaining weight and health, it is well to remember to use only those foods which are easily digested and absorbed by the body. Do not stuff yourself with so-called fattening foods, but eat smaller meals and more often. The midday, midafternoon, and before retiring refreshments are very helpful. After you have gained all the necessary pounds, you will find that you not only look much better (the thin padding of fat directly under the skin is what gives those pleasant curves to face and body) but you will also *feel* better.

Most thin people tell me they do not like fats, but when I tell them to use the delicious and easily digestible peanut oil for cooking purposes, they usually follow my advice and with excellent results.

The Chinese, for centuries, have cooked their vegetables in the most appetizing manner, in a *hot* pan, quickly, with a bit of peanut oil. Vegetables cooked in this manner seem to be most beneficial for those wishing to gain weight. Simply cut the vegetables in small bits or slices, and place them in a heavy and very hot utensil. Have a little broth or plain water steaming in the utensil and drop in the finely cut vegetables. Keep utensil covered from five to ten minutes, and let the steam tenderize the vegetables. Then add a tablespoon of peanut oil for each cup of vegetable, and sprinkle with a pinch of vegetable salt and any other flavoring you might like. Be sure that the utensil is heavy when you short-cook in this manner.

You can also make a delicious weight-gaining salad dressing with peanut oil because, more than any other oil, it can help to put on healthy pounds and curves. Take two parts of peanut oil and mix with one part of lemon juice or cider vinegar. Add a little honey, vegetable salt, garlic, or any herb of your choice. Pour this over salad greens and, finally, sprinkle with a spoonful of wheat germ. Then mix. (Reducers should take two parts of lemon juice and one part of oil.)

To help underweight people get more benefit from their meals, hot broth rather than a cold appetizer is given at the *beginning* of the meal, and hot peppermint tea is given at the *end* of the meal. The heat seems to help relax nervous and sensitive stomachs.

Then there are those wonderfully nutritious nut milks. All

nuts, especially almonds, pecans, and walnuts, are good building foods. However, most people do not chew them sufficiently, so much of their food value is lost. Fortunately, a gadget has been invented that whips nuts into a milklike consistency. You simply put one glass of your favorite fruit juice (fresh or canned) into the electric gadget. To this you add a handful of nut meats, a teaspoonful of honey, and mix. In exactly half a minute, you will have a delicious beverage with the nuts finely fletcherized and easily assimilated.

Last but not least, very ripe bananas are splendid weight-builders for thin people. They should be eaten when almost black; or you can whip a very ripe banana and a teaspoonful of honey or molasses into a glass of hot or cold milk. This is an excellent beverage to drink with meals or before retiring and it is especially helpful for "skinnies" who wish to sleep soundly.

AND HERE ARE SOME WEIGHT-GAINING MENUS TO GUIDE YOU:

BREAKFAST:
Large glass of pineapple juice
One or 2 eggs, any way but fried
Two slices of 100% whole wheat bread with butter and honey
One glass of vitamin D milk mixed with 1 tablespoon of wheat germ
If desired, café au lait with honey

MIDMORNING:
Your choice of: large glass of fortified milk, fresh pineapple juice, carrot juice, or yogurt mixed with teaspoon of brewers' yeast, molasses, and honey

LUNCH:
Cup of hot broth
Finely chopped carrot and raisin salad with fortified dressing

One whole wheat or corn muffin with honey and butter

Cup of yogurt flavored with a bit of honey or jam, if you like

Hot peppermint tea or New Orleans cup

MIDAFTERNOON: Same as midmorning, or glass of banana milk, or Curvaceous cocktail

DINNER: Finely chopped vegetable salad with yogurt dressing

Lamb roast

Sweet peas

Parsley potatoes

Sliced bananas with coconut

Peppermint tea or demitasse

BEDTIME: For deeper sleep and relaxation, your choice of: hot banana milk or glass of yogurt with teaspoon of brewers' yeast, or a cup of hot grapefruit juice with cinnamon. This is also a good time to take your calcium-vitamin D concentrate and other vitamins.

BREAKFAST: Large glass of orange juice

Cooked whole wheat cereal with honey and molasses

Whole wheat muffin with butter and honey

One glass of vitamin D milk mixed with tablespoon of wheat germ

If desired, café au lait with honey

MIDMORNING: Your choice of: large glass of fortified milk, fresh pineapple juice, carrot juice, or yogurt mixed with teaspoon of brewers' yeast, molasses, and honey

LUNCH: Cup of hot broth

Tomatoes stuffed with cottage cheese

Wheat germ muffin with butter and honey
Cup of yogurt, flavored with a bit of honey
  or jam, if you like
Hot peppermint tea or New Orleans cup

MIDAFTERNOON: Same as midmorning, or glass of banana milk,
  nut milk, or Curvaceous cocktail

DINNER: Fruit cup or hot broth
Broiled liver and bacon
Potatoes with jackets
Creamed spinach
Head lettuce with peanut oil dressing
Baked apple with cream
Peppermint tea or demitasse

BEDTIME: For deeper sleep and relaxation, your choice
  of: hot banana milk or glass of yogurt with
  teaspoon of brewers' yeast, or a cup of hot
  grapefruit juice with cinnamon. This is
  also a good time to take your calcium-
  vitamin D concentrate and other vitamins.

BREAKFAST: Large glass of apple juice
Four slices of crisp bacon, lean
Two slices 100% whole wheat bread with
  butter and honey
Glass of vitamin D milk mixed with table-
  spoon of wheat germ
If desired, café au lait

MIDMORNING: Your choice of: large glass of fortified milk,
  fresh pineapple juice, carrot juice, or yogurt mixed with teaspoon of brewers' yeast,
  molasses, and honey

LUNCH: Cup of hot broth
Creamed chicken on whole wheat toast
Fruit salad sprinkled with nuts

Cup of yogurt, flavored with a bit of honey or orange jam, if you like

Hot peppermint tea or New Orleans cup

MIDAFTERNOON: Same as midmorning, or glass of banana milk, nut milk, or Curvaceous cocktail

DINNER:

Hot broth or chopped mixed green salad
Broiled tender steak
New potatoes
Cauliflower sprinkled with American cheese
Fresh berries with honey
Peppermint tea or demitasse

BEDTIME:

For deeper sleep and relaxation, your choice of: hot banana milk or glass of yogurt with teaspoon of brewers' yeast, or a cup of hot grapefruit juice with cinnamon. This is also a good time to take your calcium-vitamin D concentrate and other vitamins.

BREAKFAST:

Large glass of orange juice
Oatmeal, Scotch style, with honey and milk
Whole wheat muffin with butter and honey
Glass of vitamin D milk mixed with tablespoon of wheat germ
If desired, café au lait

MIDMORNING:

Your choice of: large glass of fortified milk, fresh pineapple juice, carrot juice, or yogurt mixed with teaspoon of brewers' yeast, molasses, and honey

LUNCH:

Cup of hot broth
Avocado and orange salad with fortified oil dressing
Corn bread

Cup of yogurt, flavored with a bit of honey or jam, if you like

Hot peppermint tea or New Orleans cup

MIDAFTERNOON: Same as midmorning, or glass of banana milk, nut milk, or Curvaceous cocktail

DINNER:

Hot broth or Waldorf salad with wheat germ

Beef stew with potatoes

Turnip tops or spinach

Individual apple pie

Peppermint tea or demitasse

BEDTIME:

For deeper sleep and relaxation, your choice of: hot banana milk or glass of yogurt with teaspoon of brewers' yeast, or a cup of hot grapefruit juice with cinnamon. This is also a good time to take your calcium-vitamin D concentrate and other vitamins.

BREAKFAST:

Large glass of tomato juice

One or 2 eggs, any way but fried

Two slices of whole wheat toast with butter and honey

One glass of vitamin D milk mixed with tablespoon of wheat germ

If desired, café au lait

MIDMORNING: You choice of: large glass of fortified milk, fresh pineapple juice, carrot juice, or yogurt mixed with teaspoon of brewers' yeast, molasses and honey

LUNCH:

Cup of hot broth

Shrimp and celery salad with fortified oil dressing

Whole wheat muffin

Cup of yogurt, flavored with a bit of honey or jam, if you like

Hot peppermint tea or New Orleans cup

MIDAFTERNOON: Same as midmorning, or glass of banana milk, nut milk, or Curvaceous cocktail

DINNER: Hot broth, or coleslaw with yogurt dressing
Large hamburger mixed with parsley or wheat germ
Hashed brown potatoes
Short-cooked beets
Ice cream with fruit
Peppermint tea or demitasse

BEDTIME: For deeper sleep and relaxation, your choice of: hot banana milk or glass of yogurt with teaspoon of brewers' yeast, or a cup of hot grapefruit juice with cinnamon. This is also a good time to take your calcium-vitamin D concentrate and other vitamins.

BREAKFAST: Large glass of orange juice
Whole wheat pancakes or waffle with honey or maple syrup
One glass of vitamin D milk mixed with tablespoon of wheat germ
If desired, café au lait

MIDMORNING: Your choice of: large glass of fortified milk, fresh pineapple juice, carrot juice, or yogurt mixed with teaspoon of brewers' yeast, molasses and honey

LUNCH: Cup of hot broth
Large fruit salad with bananas
Two slices whole wheat cinnamon toast
One cup of yogurt, flavored with a bit of honey or jam, if you like
Hot peppermint tea or New Orleans cup

MIDAFTERNOON: Same as midmorning, or glass of banana milk, nut milk, or Curvaceous cocktail

DINNER:	Hot broth or mixed green salad Broiled fish or lobster Parsley potatoes Hot applesauce with cream and honey Peppermint tea or demitasse
BEDTIME:	For deeper sleep and relaxation, your choice of: hot banana milk or glass of yogurt with teaspoon of brewers' yeast, or a cup of hot grapefruit juice with cinnamon. This is also a good time to take your calcium-vitamin D concentrate and other vitamins.
BREAKFAST:	Large glass of pineapple juice Cooked mixed cereal (whole wheat, rye, barley, millet, etc.) with milk and molasses Muffin with butter and honey Glass of vitamin D milk mixed with tablespoon of wheat germ If desired, café au lait
MIDMORNING:	Your choice of: large glass of fortified milk, fresh pineapple juice, carrot juice, or yogurt mixed with teaspoon of brewers' yeast, molasses, and honey
LUNCH:	Cup of hot broth Two scrambled eggs with fresh stewed tomatoes on whole wheat toast Cup of yogurt flavored with a bit of honey or jam, if you like Hot peppermint tea or New Orleans cup
MIDAFTERNOON:	Same as midmorning, or glass of banana milk, nut milk, or Curvaceous cocktail
DINNER:	Hot broth or finger salad Roast chicken with dressing

Baked potato with butter
Broccoli
Sliced bananas with honey
Peppermint tea or demitasse

BEDTIME: For deeper sleep and relaxation, your choice
of: hot banana milk or glass of yogurt with
teaspoon of brewers' yeast, or a cup of hot
grapefruit juice with cinnamon. This is
also a good time to take your calcium-
vitamin D concentrate and other vitamins.

DRINK YOUR VEGETABLES

IN CZECHOSLOVAKIA is a sanatorium where peo-
ple with digestive difficulties flock by the thousands. There I
learned about the importance of fresh raw vegetable juices.
Around this sanatorium are acres and acres of vegetables, and
they are grown on rich organic soil. The head gardener and his
assistants picked golden carrots, baskets full of dark-green parsley, young tender spinach leaves, celery and celery roots. From
the orchard the men would bring ripe red apples, pears, and
other fruits of the season. The head nurse, Schwester Karoline,
would receive these vegetables and fruits with great ceremony
and a buzz would start in the diet kitchen. The vegetables were
first picked clean, then they were put into ice-cold water. Carrots
and other roots were scrubbed till they shone, and the leaves were
cleaned under running spring water. Then, with handmills, they

ground out the juices of these very fresh vegetables, and by ten o'clock every morning, each patient in the Carlsbader Sanatorium had his 8-ounce glass of fresh "live" drink of vegetable juice.

I will never forget Schwester Karoline's expression when she talked about vegetable juices. She called them the "blood of the plant." The green magic of chlorophyll, she would say, is the quickest way of healing overfed and undernourished patients. Many were English and Americans, with colitis, ulcers, liver and gall bladder difficulties. It was in this sanatorium that, more than twenty years ago, I discovered the immense healing and invigorating power of freshly made raw juices. Since then, I have recommended a daily pint of fresh vegetable juice to each and every human being I have met. And on Elizabeth Arden's Beauty Farm I made it a part of the daily beauty ritual. I am convinced, after twenty-five years, that the addition of one pint of these juices to the daily diet is one of the best safeguards against sickness and premature aging.

Needless to say, I was happy to see the excitement created all over America when Dr. Cheney of California announced that fresh cabbage juice cured ulcers in two weeks' time. His cure was based on giving his patients a quart of fresh cabbage juice or 75% cabbage and 25% celery juice. This is the first time that fresh vegetable juices were "officially recognized"—but why only cabbage juice or celery juice? All fresh juices have marvelous healing power, not only because of their vitamin and mineral content, but because of the "matière vivante" as Bircher-Benner calls it, and no chemist has yet been able to duplicate this energy. It takes the sun, soil, air, and water, Nature's mightiest forces, to produce young growing plants. No wonder the healing potential is so great in these fresh "live" juices.

For people in the second part of life, these juices are doubly

valuable because often the chewing of raw vegetables is a problem, or the raw bulk is too irritating for some. Then, of course,
much larger quantities can be taken. Not many people can eat
five large carrots, yet a grandmother of 95 can easily drink the
juice of five carrots. Then, of course, the vitamins and minerals
have been extracted from the pulp and are more easily absorbed
by the body, and there is no vitamin or mineral loss due to over-
cooking. Last, but not least, vegetable juices are delicious and
therefore the easiest and laziest way to add vitamins, minerals,
enzymes, perhaps hormones, and other as yet undiscovered factors, to the daily diet.

In England, celery juice is the great favorite. Here in America,
carrot juice comes first in popularity, then comes the more pungent celery juice, and after that the green juices of spinach, parsley, and watercress. These are rather sharp and too pungent and
should be mixed with carrot, celery, or apple juice. Also, a few
drops of lemon, orange, or pineapple juice improves the flavor. It
is very important that the health enthusiast does not defeat his
purpose. The juices must taste good, and not more than a pint a
day should be taken unless your nutritionist is treating you for
some specific cause. It is a wise habit for older people, especially
those with weakened digestion, to drink all the vegetable and fruit
juices through a straw, or better still, invest in a few glass tubes.
This prevents hasty drinking and stops unpleasant burping once
and forever.

HOW TO MAKE FRESH VEGETABLE JUICES

If you have your own garden, pick your vegetables and make
the juice as quickly as possible. In your marketing, try and go
directly to a farmer's market, and select the freshest vegetables

you can find, the younger the better; the leaves should be dark green, celery should be heavy and tender, and carrots should not be pale yellow but dark and golden. Apples should be ripe and juicy. No matter what you buy, let it be fresh. Wash everything carefully but do not soak any vegetables in water, as it will leach out vitamins B and C. Simply wash under running cold water. Do not peel carrots and other root vegetables. Simply scrub and cut in pieces small enough to fit into your vegetable juicer. If you are serious about your Look Younger, Live Longer program, invest in an electric one. They are a good investment for the entire family. There are several good ones on the market since I introduced the drinking of vegetable juices. The one I use and take with me all over the world is the easiest to operate, and I can make gallons of juice in a matter of minutes. Also, and this is important, the juices never touch tin, lead, or aluminum but pour into a bowl of metal which cannot possibly affect the color, taste, or chemistry of the juices. As soon as your vegetables are clean, work as fast as possible; put them into the juicer and drink the juice as soon as it is made. If you make extra juice, be sure to put it at once on ice and cover.

REMOVING POISONOUS SPRAYS

Some vegetable sprays are poisonous to people who lack the normal digestive acid. Also, in Mexico and the Orient, it is wise to wash all vegetables in the following solution:

Buy from your druggist one ounce of chemically pure hydrochloric acid and pour it into three quarts of water. This makes a 1 percent solution and is entirely harmless. Put this solution in an earthenware crock. It can be used for a week or more. Simply place the vegetables in the solution for five minutes; then remove and rinse with ordinary water.

GOLDEN CARROT JUICE

The dark California carrots make the most delicious juice. Drink it at once. Extra juice should be covered and refrigerated at once. Adding a few drops of orange juice will prevent the juice from losing its golden color. Drink carrot juice to your heart's content unless your waistline is out of bounds. Remember a glass of carrot juice contains about two teaspoons of sugar. Besides that, carrot juice is rich in vitamins A, B, C, and G (B_2), plus a good combination of the minerals, calcium, iron, and even iodine. Carrot juice is ideal for irritated stomachs and intestines because of the soothing vegetable mucilage it contains. Carrot juice can be mixed with practically all other juices and makes them tastier.

CARROT JUICE AND MILK

Half a cup of carrot juice and half a cup of milk makes one of the finest "builder-uppers," rich in vitamins and double rich in calcium. This combination should be adopted by all homes and sanitariums for the aged. The natural sugars will give an immediate "lift."

CELERY JUICE

Celery juice is a natural digestive and one of the best appetizers. By all means use the dark-green outside stalks. They contain more healing chlorophyll. Do not use many of the dark-green leaves; they make the juice too bitter, and they may have been sprayed. Mixing in a few drops of lemon or grapefruit juice adds to the flavor and prevents the juice from turning dark. Celery juice contains vitamins A, B, C, and some E, also the minerals sodium, potassium, and chlorine. This makes it an ideal cocktail for people with a tendency to rheumatism, and those wishing to reduce. Celery juice can be mixed with many other juices.

LIQUID APPLES

Nothing can taste better than the juice from fresh ripe apples made by cutting the unpeeled apple into four parts and putting it through a juicer. The juice cannot be compared with ordinary apple juice or cider. It should be called liquid apples because it contains the whole aroma and goodness of the apple, including vitamins A and B in fair amounts and vitamin C and G (B_2) in good amounts. Also minerals, including good amounts of sodium. Fresh apple juice has for years been recommended in gout and rheumatism, but in our program, should be drunk for its deliciousness. Here's hoping that the apple growers of the northwest install apple-juicing machines all over the land, the same as citrus growers have done. I am willing to bet that all their apples will be sold, once Americans have tasted these "liquid apples." Apple juice is mentioned here because it also blends so well with vegetable juices, and apples are plentiful the year around.

FRESH CABBAGE JUICE

Pick tender young cabbage and cut in slices to fit vegetable juicer. This makes a sweet-tasting, light-green juice, but a few dark-green stalks of celery add flavor and character to cabbage juice. It is important to make this juice tasty, since in treatment of ulcers, a whole quart of it has to be drunk daily, according to Dr. Cheney, until the ulcer is healed, which he claims takes approximately two weeks. The cabbage juice is given five times a day, a glassful in the morning, at lunch, midafternoon, at dinner, and another before retiring. All fresh vegetable juices contain vitamins A, B, and C which are important healing factors, not only vitamin U, as Dr. Cheney calls the healing factor in cabbage juice. I see no reason why cabbage juice cannot be flavored with carrot juice or any other juice which helps to eliminate the monotony of just cabbage juice. In other words, 75% cabbage juice and 25% carrot juice (or tomato juice) are bound to get the same results. Cabbage juice, as well as all other vegetable juices, must be made fresh daily and never kept from one day to the next.

SPINACH JUICE

The chlorophyll in spinach and all dark-green juices makes them valuable as potential blood-builders, but the flavor is rather sharp, so that spinach juice should be used sparingly and preferably blended with carrots and other mild-tasting vegetables. Spinach juice contains much pro-vitamin A, some vitamin B, and larger amounts of the vitamins E and G (B₂). There is also a fair amount of the minerals potassium and iodine, but the calcium is not assimilable. Equal parts of spinach, celery, and carrots make a pleasant combination.

PARSLEY JUICE

Parsley juice, from leaves and stems, makes a beautiful dark-green color, rich in chlorophyll, but like spinach juice it tastes better when blended with other vegetable juices. Parsley is really a four-star vegetable and not just a table decoration. It is the richest source of vitamin A among the vegetables, contains some B vitamin, much vitamin C, and even a small amount of vitamin E. Parsley contains many important minerals, especially iron. Make it a habit to add a bit of parsley juice to all your vegetable juice mixtures. Carrots, celery, and a bit of parsley make an ideal combination.

WATERCRESS JUICE

This dark-green liquid, like spinach and parsley juice, looks better than it tastes. You use both leaves and stems. Watercress juice contains practically all vitamins and minerals, including iodine. Therefore, a small amount fortifies other juices. Straight watercress juice, because of its sulphur content, can become an irritant and should therefore always be mixed with other juices.

LIQUID TOMATOES

Like fresh apple juice, fresh tomato juice tastes delicious. Fresh tomato juice, which is made by putting unpeeled ripe tomatoes into the juicer, bears no resemblance to the watery canned tomato juice. You will be delighted with the flavor, the color, but above all the valuable contents of this fresh juice. There is plenty of vitamin A and C, some vitamin B. Flavored with a bit of lemon and a dash of vegetable salt, it makes one of the most delicious appetizers.

FRESH PINEAPPLE JUICE

Remove the tough fibers from a ripe pineapple, and cut in slices to fit your electric juicer. The resulting foamy drink is one "fit for a duchess." Pineapple juice contains an excellent digestive called bromelin and is, therefore, most helpful before or after heavy foods are eaten. Besides bromelin, fresh pineapple juice contains the vitamins A, B, C, some G (B_2) plus nine necessary minerals including iodine. At your next dinner party, serve fresh pineapple juice flavored with a bit of watercress juice. This is the combination the Duchess of Windsor liked when I served it to her in Paris. I, therefore, dedicate this appetizer to Her Highness.

GRAPE JUICE

All fresh grapes contain the important vitamins A, B, and C plus large amounts of minerals. The large amount of inert sugar makes grapes an ideal food for elimination and reducing diets.

Thousands of tired and overweight people take the "grape cure" in Meran, Italy, and other resorts. You eat grapes to your heart's content, but the peeling and seeds are not used. You can take your own "grape cure" right at home by drinking three large glasses of fresh grape juice while grapes are in season.

GAYELORD HAUSER COCKTAIL

Cut up equal amounts of dark-green celery, golden carrots, and red apples and put through vegetable juicer. This contains practically all the vitamins, minerals, enzymes, and chlorophyll. Three glasses a day of this pleasant combination is your best life and health insurance.

COMPLEXION COCKTAIL

Peel tender young rhubarb, wash fresh ripe strawberries, and put through vegetable juicer. Two-thirds rhubarb and one-third strawberries makes a good combination. Sweeten this beautiful rose-colored juice with two teaspoons of honey. I served this combination on the beauty farm in Maine and it became very popular. This combination is mildly laxative and not more than one glassful a day should be taken.

RHUBARB AND MOLASSES

Mix one tablespoon of blackstrap molasses into a glass of fresh rhubarb juice and drink before or with breakfast. One glassful a day for two weeks makes an excellent "spring tonic" for those with liverish constitutions.

RHUBARB JUICE PROTECTS THE TEETH

In tests with orange juice, grapefruit juice, and cranberry juice, it was proved that rhubarb juice contains a protective element for the teeth. Here is a million-dollar opportunity for some enterprising manufacturer to put up fruit juices combined with a small amount of rhubarb juice, so that those with sensitive enamel need not worry about the fruit acids ruining their teeth. (Until that time, it is a wise plan to rinse the mouth thoroughly with plain water after drinking acid fruit juices.)

BEET JUICE

Scrub young beets and put through vegetable juicer. This makes an extremely beautiful wine-red juice which unfortunately tastes unpleasant. Therefore, only small amounts of beet juice should be mixed with other fruit or vegetable juices. Two-thirds of canned pineapple juice and one-third of fresh beet juice is a pleasant combination.

CUCUMBER JUICE

Cut tender unpeeled cucumbers into strips and put through vegetable juice extractor. The juice in itself is flat-tasting and must be mixed with apple juice, pineapple juice, or carrots and celery. Cucumbers are believed to have flushing action upon the kidneys, and the juice is recommended in reducing and cleansing diets. Cucumbers also contain vitamins A, B, and C, plus chlorophyll and many minerals.

LIQUID SALADS

Liquid salads are an important part of the diet therapy used at the famous Bircher-Benner clinic in Switzerland. Old and young are given two glasses of vegetable juices a day. This "liquid salad" idea is an excellent one to adopt, since many older people never masticate their salads and raw vegetables to get all the food from them. Let your imagination guide you, put any combination of vegetables into the juicer. A combination of celery, carrots, and tomatoes tastes delicious, or a combination of watercress, celery, and tomatoes. A great favorite is a mixture of celery, apples, and a bit of parsley. You might even have a "liquid salad bowl" and put head lettuce, a bit of cabbage, celery, a small cucumber, tomatoes, and half a green peper through the extractor. Flavor with a bit of vegetable salt and a few drops of lemon. Such a liquid salad taken before a meal is a wonderful way of breaking yourself away from overrich salad dressing.

THE ONE DAY REST CURE

YEARS AGO I searched for a way to make up for our dietetic carelessness, and other carelessness, such as lack of sleep, lack of relaxation, because sooner or later all our extravagances leave their imprints on our bodies and faces. I came to the conclusion that the best way to make up for such losses is to declare one day out of every week a health holiday, a rest cure, and to give one day to our Look Younger, Live Longer regime. Everybody knows that, after a day of rest, both body and spirit are lighter and brighter, and for that reason yearly vacations have become a national good habit; but two weeks or even a month every year is not enough in these days of "high tension" living. Why wait until you are so exhausted that you cannot relax and let go on your vacation? There is good scientific reasoning that smaller and more frequent meals are better for busy people, and over a period of thirty years, I have become convinced that short and more frequent rest periods are health-giving and prolong our youthfulness. Give yourself this one day a week rest cure. Make it any day in the week, or Sunday if that is your only day away from the job, but go all the way. Not only does the brain need a rest but the entire man needs a rest; especially, the "inner man" needs a holiday from overeating.

On this day, be as lazy as possible, stay in bed as long as you like, shut off the telephone and talk as little as possible (if women only knew how much energy is wasted through idle chit-chat and gossip, they'd stop at once). In other words, this is your day to relax—relax, let go of all tension. See your lesson on relaxation and take the Body Slant two or three times during the day; it's your chance to stop that constant downward pull. This is probably the laziest, best, and easiest of all exercises. Just lie there, be alone in your room and rest your weary bones. Let go, and as you lie there you might as well use one of the simplest and most wonderful forces to youthify the body—breathe, breathe, breathe slowly and gently, breathe in through your nose, then slowly, and a little more forcefully, breathe out through the mouth. Do this for three minutes three times a day, or whenever you are relaxing. Remember that every time you breathe in, you are breathing in life-prolonging oxygen; and when you are breathing out, you are expelling waste. But what is more important for you, and this is not wishful thinking, every time you breathe in you are giving a gentle massage to your heart, arteries, lungs, and intestines, and every cell of the body receives the benefit of this increased amount of fresh air. Even your eyes will be better and, if you have dark circles under your eyes, they will become less and less noticeable and finally disappear. Here is hoping that all health clubs, beauty farms, and institutions adopt and use this simple, consciously controlled form of deep, slow rhythmic breathing. It is by far the best exercise to prevent the inner organs from premature aging. I also hope that all intelligent men and women, especially those who work under tension, will occasionally stop and do a few rhythmic breaths during their working hours. The celebrated Professor Tirala has demonstrated in hundreds of cases that tension and high blood pressure can be corrected by deep, slow rhythmic breathing. So I urge you, on this your One Day Rest Cure, to let go and breathe in as much fresh air as possible; nothing is as helpful to clear one's brain and revive one's spirit.

Your menu for this *gesundheits-tag* should be light, to give an overworked digestive tract a rest. You will overeat the vitamin-rich, mineral-rich, easy-to-digest foods, and you will under-eat the hard-to-digest, high acid, and fattening foods for *just one day*. Your "inner man," which includes your stomach, liver, and gall bladder, and 28 feet of abused intestines, will have a day *off!* This is an easy diet to follow; even weak sisters and over-eaters in general can follow it with ease. You may be cheating your appetite, but your "inner man" is having a feast of vitamins, minerals, enzymes, easy-to-digest proteins—and the result will be that you look better and feel better the very next day.

If I can inspire you to make this one-day-a-week rest cure part of your busy life, I know that you will be as enthusiastic about it as are thousands of my students all over the world. And here, sir or madame, is your menu to choose from:

> fresh fruits, fruit juices, fresh vegetables, salads, liquid salads, yogurt, cottage cheese, buttermilk, molasses and honey.

> hot beverages: peppermint tea, papaya tea, strawberry tea, fortified milk, Modern Coffee, New Orleans cup.

And this is how it can be arranged. Remember to stay in bed as long as you like—pamper yourself. Let your husband, your mother-in-law, or your maid bring you a glass of freshly squeezed orange or grapefruit juice or fortified tomato juice—as much as you like—and drink it through a straw. Now go and snooze some more, even if you do not sleep. Just lie there as relaxed and carefree as a rag doll, breathe slowly and deeply for three minutes, don't answer the telephone, and above all don't talk. Be a miser with your energy *one* day a week.

BREAKFAST: Whenever you want it—your choice: peppermint tea, papaya tea, strawberry tea, New Orleans cup, Modern Coffee sweetened with molasses or honey (no cream today, let the gall bladder rest).

MIDMORNING: If hungry during the morning—your choice: fortified tomato juice or sauerkraut and tomato juice (half and half) or celery juice or carrot juice or liquid salad or fortified milk

LUNCHEON: Any time you like—you are no slave to time today:
Hot clear broth or liquid salad
Large salad
Your choice of: any fresh vegetables, chopped very fine, with yogurt dressing (the finer you chop it the less work for the "inner man"), or sauerkraut salad sprinkled with lemon and caraway seeds, or glass of yogurt flavored with molasses and honey
Hot beverage, as for breakfast

MIDAFTERNOON: Same as midmorning, or hot tea with lemon —try some of the fragrant herb teas

DINNER:

Liquid salad or hot broth

Four tablespoons fresh cottage cheese sprinkled with chives or parsley or green onions or caraway seeds (a bit of lemon if desired), or large finely chopped carrot salad with half-cup thick yogurt dressing

Beverage: your choice of: fortified milk, yogurt, herb tea, New Orleans cup or demitasse

BEDTIME

So there is no possible chance of cheating your body of any of the important vitamins or minerals, fortify yourself with 1 fish liver oil capsule for vitamin A and D, 1 tablet of ascorbic acid for vitamin C, 1 wheat germ oil capsule for vitamin E, and drink down with a cup of fortified hot milk flavored with a teaspoon each of blackstrap molasses and brewers' yeast for vitamin B and more protein.

Here's hoping you took the Body Slant and that you relaxed and breathed deeply for a few minutes, at least. If so, you can say good night to your conscience and fall into *deep* sleep—no dreams tonight! I recommend this one day rest cure to all busy executives, and dedicate it to Mr. and Mrs. Eddie Rickenbacker who for years have thrived on my diets.

THE ONE DAY HOLLYWOOD LIQUID DIET

Y OU HAVE probably heard that many of the Hollywood glamour ladies and handsome men are in constant fear of being overweight, and that the camera not only exaggerates their weight, but shows tiredness and dissipation which even clever make-up cannot cover. For that reason, many of the stars declare a health holiday, stay at home, lie in the sun and, for an entire day, sip only liquids. This is a good plan for all those who feast and celebrate too much; or for whenever the waistline feels a bit tight. It is also a wise plan to follow for those who "eat out" a great deal and really never get enough of the fresh vitamin-rich fruits and vegetables. However, one gets much hungrier on an all-liquid diet than on the One Day Rest Cure Diet, so I recommend the all-liquid diet only to the experienced dieters.

It's actually very simple to carry out. Make it a day of rest for mind and body, stay in bed longer, leave the windows wide open; do some slow, deep breathing, inhale gently through the nose, exhale more forcefully through the mouth. Remember that besides inhaling the most necessary element, oxygen, you give the heart, aorta, and lungs a gentle massage. If possible, be as elegant as the movie stars; rest all day. Have someone wait on you who will serve you the juices absolutely fresh. Drink them immediately and through a straw or glass tube. Why, you ask? Because the juices will agree with you better; you mix them better with saliva and you don't gulp them down. That's when they disagree with you. And here is how you can take a "juice day" any time you feel the need for it:

BREAKFAST:	Your choice: 1 large glass of orange juice or grapefruit juice or fortified tomato juice Two cups hot peppermint tea or 2 cups hot papaya tea sweetened with honey or 1 cup black coffee or café au lait
MIDMORNING:	Your choice: large glass of celery juice or carrot juice or apple juice. If no fresh vegetable juices are available, drink fresh fruit juice.
LUNCHEON:	Your choice: 2 cups Hauser broth or 1 glass yogurt flavored with cinnamon or nutmeg or honey Hot beverage as for breakfast
MIDAFTERNOON:	Same as midmorning, or tea with lemon, or fortified milk
DINNER:	Hauser Broth or liquid salad One glass of yogurt flavored with honey or grated orange rind Beverage: papaya-mint tea or demitasse
BEDTIME:	Check up on your elimination; if necessary take an herbal laxative. Also take vitamins A and D, C, and E, and drink down with a glass of hot milk fortified with molasses.

I recommend this one day liquid diet to all who want to give the "inner man" an occasional rest. I dedicate this diet to Walter Pidgeon, who long ago received such amazing benefits from my diets.

SPECIAL BUILDING DIET BEFORE OR
AFTER SURGERY

*T*HERE IS MUCH that diet can do to speed up healing after operations or tooth extractions. The time at the hospital can be cut considerably and the discomfort and suffering can be greatly relieved. To help digestion and absorption at such trying times, it is wise to restrict the diet to soft, easily digested foods and give small but frequent meals. I also recommend such a diet to all the grossmamas and grosspapas wherever they are. I realize that this diet is very different from the present hospital diet, but in this atomic age, with changes all around us, our hospitals must also change with the times. I respectfully dedicate this special building diet to all the dietitians in all the hospitals everywhere!

7:00 a.m.   Fortified warm milk or Milk Lassie

8:30 a.m.   Half cup wheat germ cooked as a cereal, served with milk and honey
One slice 100% whole wheat, if desired
Fish liver oil capsule supplying at least 25,000 units of vitamin A; vitamin C tablet, 100 milligrams; vitamin E capsule, 30 milligrams; enzyme tablet, if digestion poor

10:30 a.m. One glass fortified milk and blackstrap molasses

12:30 p.m. One cup vegetable cream soup finely fletcherized in electric mixer
One thin slice wheat germ bread
Fortified yogurt with honeyed fruit
Vitamin C tablet, 100 milligrams
Enzyme tablet, if digestion poor

345

3:00 p.m.   Glass of pineapple, grapefruit, or tomato juice fortified
with 1 tablespoon dried brewers' yeast

5:30 p.m.   Omelet or soufflé or broiled liver
One fortified potato
Two tablespoons mashed or puréed but short-cooked
vegetable

8:30 p.m.   One glass fortified milk and blackstrap molasses

10:00 p.m. Hot milk and 2 calcium tablets

When the above plan is used, the physician can add even more
nutrients, depending entirely on the individual case. Large
amounts of vitamin B help the process of elimination and prevent the horror of horrors—gas pains. Calcium and more calcium
decreases the chances of hemorrhaging, and vitamin C and more
vitamin C shortens the healing time and helps to prevent those
ugly large scars.

THOSE ATOMIC AMINO ACIDS

AMINO ACID MOLECULES are small and contain
from ten to thirty-five atoms! It took exactly one hundred years of
research for this momentous discovery; a discovery as vital for the
good of man as the atomic bomb can be for the destruction of
man. Another great victory of this hundred-year research is the
discovery that only eight of the twenty amino acids are necessary
for health and longer life. The other twelve can be manufactured
by the body. And now, before you wonder what this is all about,

let me say that all first class protein foods are made up from and contain these amino acids. So it is for a very good scientific reason that I recommend larger amounts of fortified milk, lean meat, eggs, cheese, yeast, and the unappreciated soya bean in the Live Longer Diet. All these are first class proteins and contain the best source of amino acids. The names of the eight essential amino acids may sound strange, but in years to come you will hear a great deal about them, so let me be the first to introduce you to:

Lysine	Phenylalanine
Leucine	Threonine
Isoleucine	Methionine
Tryptophan	Valine.

Don't be confused by these strange-sounding names, just remember that all of these are obtained in first class proteins. Also remember that you have to have enough protein foods each and every day. If not, the body takes the proteins from the muscles to keep the heart, the liver and other essential organs in good condition. When this happens, the body ages fast and furious as thousands of victims of concentration camps proved—old, decrepit-looking people because of protein starvation. The average man should eat not less than 70 grams of protein, the average woman not less than 60 grams each and every day. This is the most expensive item especially for people with large families. For that reason, I recommend the fortification of ordinary foods with dried skim milk, an inexpensive source of good protein, as well as brewers' yeast, wheat germ and soya products. Before or after surgery, in burns, ulcers and kidney difficulties, your doctor will recommend extra amounts of first class proteins which contain all of those eight atomic amino acids. Here is a list of protein foods.

Use it to check your protein intake until you have formed the habit of eating not less than 60 to 70 grams a day for the rest of your life.

PROTEIN FOODS:	AMOUNT	GRAMS OF PROTEIN
Beef	Average helping	17
Chicken	Average helping	18
Heart	Average helping	11
Kidney	Average helping	11
Lamb chop	1 medium	10
Liver	Average helping	19
Steak	Average helping	21
Turkey	Average helping	21
Milk, whole	1 qt.	30
Milk, dried skim	½ cup	53
Yogurt	1 qt.	33
Cheese	1 piece, 2x1x1 inches	12
Cottage cheese	3 tbsp.	10
Cream cheese	1½ tbsp.	8
Egg	1	6
Salmon, canned	1/3 cup	22
Tuna fish, canned	2 tbsp.	12
Shrimp	6 medium	8
Peanuts	2 tbsp.	10
Peanut flour	1 cup	59
Peanut butter	2 tbsp.	14
Walnuts	½ cup	8
Pecans	10 meats	3
Lima beans	½ cup	8
Navy beans	½ cup	6
Soybeans, dried	½ cup	51
Soya flour	1 cup	37
Lentils	½ cup	9
Peas, dried	½ cup	7

PROTEIN FOODS:	AMOUNT	GRAMS OF PROTEIN
Barley, whole	½ cup cooked	8
Buckwheat, whole	1/3 cup	12
Rice, brown	¾ cup	3
Shredded wheat	1 biscuit	3
Wheat germ	½ cup	24
Yeast, dried	1 tbsp.	4

MORE VITAMINS FOR LONGER LIFE

NOT FEWER but more vitamins are necessary in the second part of life. Dr. H. C. Sherman, in his longevity experiments, pointed out again and again that the ideal intake would be four times the maintenance amount, which means optimum amounts as I suggest in all the menus. Let me give you here not the boring details but the highlights of the vitamins most important to our Look Younger, Live Longer plan.

You need more VITAMIN A for brighter eyes, better skin, more resistance to disease, longer life. Consequences of insufficient vitamin A are: burning eyes, night blindness, rough skin, kidney stones, stony deposits on teeth, risk of infection.

Best sources of this vitamin: chiefly animal foods, fish liver oils, liver, kidneys, butter, cream, milk. Vitamn A is also manufactured by the liver from all green and yellow fruits and vegetables.

For a longer and healthier life, fortify yourself daily with

10,000, or still better, 20,000 units. Select from the following list:

Very Best Sources	Amount	Units
Fish liver oil	1 capsule	25,000
Kale	⅞ cup	17,500
Liver (calf)	8 oz.	12,590
Broccoli	2/3 cup	10,800
Turnip greens	1 cup	10,000
Spinach	¾ cup	9,375
Collards	2/3 cup	7,000
Potatoes, sweet	1 medium	5,250
Squash, Hubbard	⅞ cup	5,000

Good Sources		
Pumpkin	¾ cup	3,000
Apricots	2 whole	2,880
Carrots	¾ cup	2,520
Peaches, yellow	2 halves	1,400
Prunes	5 fruit	1,250
Tomatoes	1 whole	1,250
Kidney, lamb	4 oz.	1,150
Beans, green	¾ cup	750
Peas, green	½ cup	750
Butter	2 tbsp.	720
Cantaloupe	½	600
Asparagus	6 6-inch stalks	325
Cheese, Cheddar	1½x1½x1¼ inches	500
Corn, yellow	1 8-inch ear	500
Egg	1	500
Soybeans, fresh	½ cup	150

THE IMPORTANT VITAMIN B FAMILY

Each year the prolific vitamin B family becomes more important. There are about 20 members, and each one plays some specific part in health and long life. Most people take vitamin B₁ because it gives added energy and helps a tired heart. But it is a much wiser plan to include all the different members of the complex and, whenever possible, to obtain your vitamin B in natural food form. In that way, you obtain the benefit of all the different food factors. That is why our Live Longer menus contain such generous amounts of the richest natural sources of all the B vitamins.

You need more vitamin B₁ for better digestion, healthy nerves, healthy heart. Consequences of insufficient vitamin B₁ are: constipation, poor digestion, tiredness, nervousness, heart trouble, insomnia, neuritis, gas.

Best sources of this vitamin: brewers' yeast, wheat germ, corn germ, blackstrap molasses, powdered skim milk, whole grains, and yogurt which manufactures vitamin B in the intestines. Here is a list of vitamin B₁ foods. Check and see how much of this important vitamin you have obtained in the last 24 hours. For a longer life, I recommend 4 to 6 milligrams a day, or more:

Very Best Sources	Amount	Milligrams
Brewers' yeast	1 tablespoon	2.25
Brewers' yeast	4 tablets	2.25
Wheat germ	½ cup	2.60
Cottonseed flour	1 cup	1.18
Rice bran	¼ cup	1.12
Dried skim milk	½ cup	0.55
Whole wheat flour	1 cup	0.4

RIBOFLAVIN, second member of the B family, is the vitamin which Dr. Sherman says is especially essential for long life. Laboratory animals outlive their normal life span by 10 percent when it is generously added to their diet. This factor is also of great importance because it helps the eyes. Even cataracts are being stopped by its use. Nutritionists recommend as much as 15 milligrams of riboflavin a day, plus all other vitamins and 3 tablespoons of brewers' yeast. Riboflavin, plus vitamin A, is also needed to prevent night blindness. The average adult should be sure to obtain 5 milligrams of riboflavin each and every day. Here are some foods you may select:

Very Best Sources	Amount	Milligrams
Dried skim milk	½ cup	2.61
Brewers' yeast	1 tablespoon	1.00
Milk (fresh)	1 quart	2.00
Beef liver	2 slices	2.00
Wheat germ	½ cup	0.75

NIACIN, third member of the vitamin B family, is now called niacin amide. It is necessary for healthy skin, healthy blood, and good digestion. Here are the foods richest in niacin: wheat germ, dried skim milk, brewers' yeast, whole wheat flour, molasses, soya flour.

PYRIDOXINE, or vitamin B_6, is gaining a great deal of importance because it helps to relax nervous, twitchy, and sleepless people. Most middle-aged people do not obtain sufficient pyridoxine and, since it is expensive, most vitamin formulas contain too little. Foods containing this important vitamin are: wheat germ, brewers' yeast, egg yolk, milk, and liver.

PANTOTHENIC ACID almost became a "glamour" vitamin because it is involved in the graying of the hair. It proved disappointing, however, since many other factors enter into the graying of the hair. Pantothenic acid is important because it does help prevent old-age changes, especially when combined with another member of the vitamin B family. Here are some foods that contain good amounts of pantothenic acid: blackstrap molasses, peanuts, brewers' yeast, dried milk, liver, egg yolk, kidneys, wheat germ, whole wheat cereal.

PARA-AMINOBENZOIC ACID is necessary for the normal functioning of the glands and is also valuable for the prevention of gray hair. The best foods containing para-aminobenzoic acid are: liver, rice bran, brewers' yeast, blackstrap molasses.

FOLIC ACID has made headlines since it has been used successfully in pernicious anemia. It also plays some part in retaining normal hair coloring. The best foods containing folic acid are: yeast, liver.

INOSITOL is important for the stimulation of hair growth. Foods containing inositol are: fruits, nuts, whole grains, milk, yogurt, yeast, meat.

BIOTIN is needed for energy production and promotes mental health so necessary for the second part of life. Best biotin foods are: egg yolk (not white), liver, yeast, yogurt, tomatoes, kidneys.

CHOLIN helps to keep the liver healthy, digests fats, and assists the gall bladder functioning. It is found in: brewers' yeast, liver.

And so ends a short family history of the vitamin B complex, as it is known today. There are still other members not yet completely understood. And this is the very reason why you should take your vitamins, whenever possible, in some natural food because then, and then only, are you sure of obtaining all the food factors, discovered and undiscovered. If you have studied the list of the vitamin B family, you, too, will be impressed with the importance of our simple and inexpensive wonder foods: brewers' yeast, liver, powdered milk, wheat germ, blackstrap molasses. Make these a part of your daily living.

You need more VITAMIN C for healthy gums, pliant joints, young connective tissue, vital resistance. Consequences of insufficient vitamin C are: bleeding gums, rheumatism, stiffness, troublesome veins and arteries, brittle bones, susceptibility to all infections.

Best sources of this vitamin: fresh citrus fruits, red and green peppers, canned fruit and vegetable juices.

For keeping the body young and pliant, use 15,000 to 20,000 units of vitamin C each and every day.

Very Best Sources	Amount	Units
Broccoli	2/3 cup	2,400
Kale	7/8 cup	2,185
Liver, calves', beef, or lamb	8 oz.	1,725
Cauliflower	1 cup	1,500
Cantaloupe	½	1,200
Mustard greens	1 cup	1,200
Peppers, red	1 3-inch piece	1,150
Spinach	1½ cups	1,125
Strawberries	¾ cup	1,000
Brussel sprouts	1 cup	1,000
Grapefruit	½ cup	850
Cabbage	1 cup	845
Orange	1 medium	800
Pineapple	1 cup	750
Turnips	¾ cup	720
Beet greens	1 cup	700
Collards	2/3 cup	700

Very Best Sources	Amount	Units
Peppers, green	1 3-inch piece	677
Soybeans, green	½ cup	600
Turnip greens	1 cup	600
Parsnips	¾ cup	540
Tomato	1	475
Lima beans, green	½ cup	450
Asparagus	6 6-inch stalks	432
Potatoes, sweet	1 medium	425
Endive	½ cup	400
Sardine	1 large	360
Avocado	½	340
Peaches, yellow	1	281

You need more VITAMIN D for good teeth, better relaxation, sound nerves, better sleep. Consequences of insufficient vitamin D are: poor bone structure, bad teeth, nervous tension, calcium deficiency, arthritis, nearsightedness.

Best source of this vitamin: the sunshine, if you can relax in it for two hours each day. Otherwise: fish liver oil, cod liver oil, halibut liver oil, irradiated yeast. This vitamin is toxic; not more than 5,000 units should be taken each day unless supervised by your physician.

You need more VITAMIN E for your heart, your muscles, painless menopause, good skin, normal sex life. Consequences of insufficient vitamin E are: heart trouble, muscular atrophy, female difficulties.

Best sources of vitamin E: fresh wheat germ, wheat germ oil, corn oil, green lettuce, avocados.

VITAMIN K is needed for normal blood coagulation. The speed with which blood clots after surgery depends on the amount of vitamin K in the body. Fortunately, there are many foods containing vitamin K: all green leaves as spinach, beet tops, Swiss chard, but especially the green tops of carrots.

You need more VITAMIN P for healthy veins and arteries, normal blood pressure, prevention of strokes. Consequences of insufficient vitamin P are: broken veins, hemorrhages, high blood pressure, porous blood vessels.

Best sources of this vitamin: green peppers, citrus fruit, especially lemon and orange peel. To make vitamin P extract, see page 285.

MORE MINERALS FOR LONGER LIFE

MINERALS are just as important to a longer life as vitamins. In fact, they work together. Thousands of misinformed people take their vitamins conscientiously, but neglect the less glamorous minerals. There are 16 or more minerals essential to good health and vitality, but here I shall describe only those which are important for a Look Younger, Live Longer plan. (For information about other minerals, see *Diet Does It.*)

You need more *CALCIUM* for good posture, stronger bones and teeth, normal nerve action, rhythmic heart, good nails. Consequences of insufficient calcium are: bad posture, tooth decay, brittle bones, nervousness, cramps, nervous heart, nervous headaches.

Best sources of calcium: powdered skim milk, whole milk,

cheese, but especially yogurt and buttermilk because the calcium dissolves easier in lactic acid. Drink a pint, or still better, a quart of some form of milk each day and add years to your life and life to your years.

You need PHOSPHORUS for building and maintaining good bones and teeth, for all glandular secretions, for vital energy. Consequences of insufficient phosphorus are: tooth decay, susceptibility to pyorrhea, easily broken bones.

Best sources of phosphorus: milk, cheese, egg yolks, meat, fish, whole cereals, peas, and beans. Please remember that calcium and phosphorus are utilized in the body *only* when vitamin D is present.

You need more IRON for a rosy complexion, more pep, better memory, warmer hands and feet. Consequences of insufficient iron are: anemia, tiredness, forgetfulness, lack of endurance.

Best sources of iron: liver, blackstrap molasses, apricots, eggs, oysters. In case of anemia, nutritionists recommend concentrated iron salts as ferrous mucate or ferrous chloride, in tablet form.

You need IODINE for more stamina, greater endurance, healthy thyroid gland, keeping slim. Consequences of insufficient iodine are: goiter, overweight, tiredness, menopausal difficulties, mental depressions.

Best sources of iodine: all fish from the oceans, all sea vegetation as kelp, sea moss, sea lettuce, sea greens, fresh or in dried form. All salt used in cooking or at table should be iodized, and already thousands of my students are using an iodized vegetable salt that gives them small amounts of organic iodine every time they salt their food.

REFERENCES AND SUGGESTED READING

Behr, Valentin *Arterien Verkalkung*. Hannover: Wilkens Verlag, 193

Berman, Louis *The Glands Regulating Personality*. New York: Macmillan Co., 1928
Food and Character. New York: Houghton, Mifflin Co., 1932.
New Creations in Human Beings. Garden City, N. Y.: Doubleday, Doran and Co., 1938

Best, C. H. and Ridout, J. H. Choline as a dietary factor. *Ann. Rev. Biochem.* (1947) 8, 349.

Bircher-Benner *Früchtespeisen and Rohgemüse*. Zurich, 1936.

Bogert, Jean L. *Nutrition and Physical Fitness*. Philadelphia: W. B. Saunders Co., 1949.

Bogomolets, Alexander A. *The Prolongation of Life*. New York: Duell, Sloan and Pearce, 1946.

Brandaleone, H. E. and Steele, J. M. Effect of pantothenic acid and para-aminobenzoic acid on gray hair in humans. *Proc. Soc. Exper. Biol. Med.*, (1943) 43, 1331.

Brande, Dorothea *Wake Up and Live!* New York: Simon & Schuster, 1936

Brauchle, Alfred *Naturheilkunde* Leipzig: Reclam., 1938.

Brentano, Lowell *Ways to Better Hearing*. New York: Franklin Watts Inc., 1946

Carnegie, Dale *How To Stop Worrying and Start Living*. New York: Simon & Schuster, 1948.

Cooper, Berber, and Mitchell *Nutrition in Health and Disease*. Philadelphia: J. B. Lippincott Co., 1948.

Council on Foods and Nutrition. The Harmful Effects of Mineral Oil. *J. Am. Med. Assn.*, (1943) 123,967.

Cowley, Gail *Over Seventy*. Boston: Meador Press, 1944.

Davis, Adelle *Let's Cook It Right*. New York: Harcourt, Brace, 1947.
Vitality Through Planned Nutrition. New York: Macmillan Co., 1949. 2nd Ed.

Davis, Hallowell *Hearing and Deafness*. New York: Murray Hill Books, 1947.

Dyer, H. C., and Roe, J. H. The relation of nutrition to gastric function. *Am. J. Digest. Dis.*, (1943)15,189

Eddy, W. H., and Dalldorf, G. *The Avitaminoses*. Baltimore: Williams & Wilkins Co., 1948.

Eller, J. J., and Diaz, L. A. Vitamins for gray hair. *N. Y. State J. Med.* (1943) 53, 47.

Fink, David Harold *Release From Nervous Tension*. New York: Simon & Schuster, 1943.

Goldziehier, Max A. *The Endocrine Glands*. New York: Appleton-Century, 1939.

Graupner, Heinz *Hormone und Vitamine*. Berlin: Deutscher Verlag, 1940.

Halle, Albert *Kunst und Wissenschaft Des Essens*. Berlin: Weiner Verlag, 1934.

Hauser, Gayelord *Diet Does it*. New York: Coward McCann, 1944.
The Gayelord Hauser Cook Book. ibid., 1946.
Eat and Grow Beautiful. London: Faber and Faber, Ltd., 1936.
Manger Pour Etre Belles. Paris: Libraire Arthène Fayard, 1937.
Dictionary of Foods. Tempo Books, Inc. 1934.

Food Science and Health. ibid., 1935.

Better Eyes Without Glasses. London: Faber and Faber Ltd., 1941.

Hickman, K. C. The sparing action of vitamin E on vitamin A and carotene. *J. Biol. Chem.*, (1944) 152, 303, 313, 321.

Horney, Karen *Our Inner Conflicts.* New York: W. W. Norton, 1946.

Hovey, Sallie *The Rehabilitation of Eve.* Chicago: Hyman, McGee Co., 1924.

Hunt, A. H. The role of vitamin C in healing. *Brit. J. Surg.* (1941) 28, 436.

Jackson, Josephine A. and Salisbury, Helen M. *Outwitting Our Nerves.* Garden City Publishing Co., 1944.

Joliffe, N. Treatment of psychiatric disorders with vitamins. *J. Am. Med. Assn.* (1941) 117, 1948.

Vitamins and Hormones. Ithaca: Cornell University Press, 1943.

Lawton, George *Aging Successfully.* New York: Columbia University Press, 1946.

New Goals for Old Age. ibid., 1943.

Linke, A. Adolphe *A Study in Reconstructive Mental Hygiene.* Boston: Meador Publishing Co., 1939.

Lohner, Viktor *Mensch und Heilpflanze.* Linz-Donau: Pirngruber Verlag, 1941

McLester, James S. *Nutrition and Diet in Health and Disease.* Philadelphia: W. B. Saunders Co., 1949.

Martin, Lillien J. *A Handbook For Old Age Counsellors.* San Francisco: Geertz Printing Co., 1944.

Mellanby, E. Influence of vitamins and hormones on physiology and pathology. *Proc. Roy. Soc. Med.* (1943) 26, 621.

Morgan, A. F., and Simms, H. D. Senescence produced by vitamin deficiency. *Science* (1939) 89, 565.

Nutrition Reviews Diet and hypertension. (1948) 6, 293.
Nutrition and arthritis. (1949) 7, 33.
Nutrition in diabetes. (1948) 6, 257.
Nutrition in endocrinology. (1949) 7, 97.

Overstreet, H. A. *The Mature Mind.* New York: W. W. Norton, 1949.

Owens, L. B., Wright, J. and Brown, E. Vitamins in the treatment of diabetes. *Am. J. Med. Sci.* (1941) 201, 636.

Pitkin, Walter M. *The Best Years.* New York: A. A. Wyn, 1946.

Price, Weston A. *Nutrition and Physical Degeneration.*

Ray, Marie Beynon. *How Never To Be Tired.* Indianapolis: Bobbs, Merrill Co., 1944.
How to Conquer Your Handicaps. ibid., 1948.

Rorty, James and Norman, N. Philip *Tomorrow's Food.* New York: Prentice-Hall Inc., 1947.

Roemheld, Ludwig *Wie Verlaengere Ich Mein Leben.* Stuttgart: Enke Verlag, 1941.

Saint-Pierre, Dr. *Prolonger La Vie.* Paris: Champrosay, 1948.

Sherman, Henry C. *Selected Works.* New York: Macmillan Co., 1948.

Shute, E. V., Shute, W. E., and Vogelsang, A. B. Vitamin E in the treatment of heart disease. *Med. Rec.* (1947) 160, 279.

Spies, T. D. Pantothenic acid and human nutrition. *J. Am. Med. Assn.* (1940) 115, 523.
Nutrition and Rehabilitation.

Spink, W. W. Vitamin C and immunity. *J. Immunol.* (1942) 44, 289.

Strauss, Eduard *Die Heilmittel.* Hamburg: Froehlich Verlag, 1949.

Taylor, R. D. Effects of large doses of vitamins in hypertensive patients. *Am. J. Med. Sci.* (1943) 206, 659.

Tirala, Lothar *Heilung Des Blutdrucks Durch Atemübungen.* Bern: Alpha Verlag, 1949

Vischer, A. L. *Old Age—Its Compensations and Rewards.* New York: Macmillan Co., 1947.

Von Hesse, Elizabeth Ferguson. *So To Speak.* Philadelphia: J. B. Lippincott Co., 1941.

Voronoff, Serge *The Sources of Life.* Boston: Bruce Humphries, Inc., 1943.

Warfield, Frances *Cotton In My Ears.* New York: Viking Press, 1948.

Weitzel, Willy *Das Raetsel Des Pflanzenblutes.* Dresden: Pahl, 1934.

Wolbach, S. B. Vitamin A deficiency and the nervous system. *Arch. Path.* (1941) 32,689.

Wrench, G. T. *The Wheel of Health.* Milwaukee: Lee Foundation for Nutritional Research, 1945.

Zimmerman, F. T., Burgemeister, B. B., and Putnam, T. J. Glutamic acid and intelligence. *Am. J. Psychiat.* (1948) 104, 593.

Acknowledgment is made to the following magazines: *Vitamin News, Diet Digest, Newsweek, Magazine Digest, Best Years, Coronet, Hippokrates, Wendepunkt, Je Sais Tout, Sapere.*

INDEX

INDEX

Abdomen, flattening of, 192; strengthening of, 18, 127–130
Absent-mindedness, 76–77
A.C.S. (see Antireticulae cytotoxic serum)
Acidity, natural, 45–46
Acidophilus milk, 13
Acids, and red blood, 165
Acrolein, 287
Activities, balancing of, 219–221
Adenine, 74
Adrenalin, 93
Adrenals, 93
Adult education courses, 206, 226, 233
Africa, cancer in, 64
After All, 211
Age, 10, 17, 21; attributes of, 202; examples of, 206–209; and wrinkles, 166–167 (See also Middle age; Old age)
Agelessness, 116–117, 228; and calcium, 132; in clothes, 195; and relaxation, 123, 126; secret of, 209, 213–214
"Aging Successfully," 233
Air bath, 189
Alcoholics, 98–99, 101–102
Alcoholics Anonymous, 99, 102
Alexandra, Queen, of Yugoslavia, 276
Alkalizers, 45–46
All-in-one cocktail, 264–265
Allergies, 80; and calcium, 92; food, 79; and nutrition, 78
Almonds, 276
Alpha tocopherol (see Vitamin E)
Alton, 60

American Fashion Show, first, 146–147
American Geriatrics Society, 59, 146
American Hearing Society, 138, 141, 143
American Journal of Surgery (New York), 66
American Medical Association, 204; *Journal,* 50, 242
Amino acids, 23, 28, 45, 53–54, 70, 77, 81, 96, 121, 134, 155, 263, 346–347
Ammonia, and tooth decay, 149
Anemia, 70–72; blood test for, 71; low-protein, 71; menopausal, 85; pernicious, 71–72
Anger, 219
Angina pectoris, 37–38
Animals, laboratory, cancer in, 64–65; and kidney stones, 67
Antireticular cytotoxic serum (A.C.S.), 13
Apoplexy, 59–61
Appetites, training of, 106
Apple juice, 251, 264, 290
Apples, liquid, 333
Applesauce, five-minute, 273, 282–283
Apricot juice, 264
Apricot whip, 283
Apricots, 134, 164, 281
Aptitude tests, 221
Arden, Elizabeth, 127, 283; beauty farm, 145, 162, 170, 240, 301, 329 (See also Main Chance Beauty Farm)
Arginine, 96–97

367